Biosynthetic Products for Cancer Chemotherapy

Volume 1

Biosynthetic Products for Cancer Chemotherapy

Volume 1

George R. Pettit
Arizona State University, Tempe

PLENUM PRESS · NEW YORK AND LONDON

Library of Congress Cataloging in Publication Data

Pettit, George R
  Biosynthetic products for cancer chemotherapy.

  Bibliography: p.
  Includes index.
    1. Cancer—Chemotherapy. 2. Antineoplastic agents. I. Title [DNLM: 1. Neo-
plasms—Drug therapy. 2. Antineoplastic agents. QZ267 P511b]
RC271.C5P47   616.9'94'061   76-54146
ISBN 0-306-37687-3 (v. 1)

© 1977 Plenum Press, New York
A Division of Plenum Publishing Corporation
227 West 17th Street, New York, N.Y. 10011

Printed in the United States of America

*To the far-sighted, enlightened and dedicated
present and past members of the National Cancer Institute
whose great contributions and personal sacrifice have
provided a firm basis for cancer chemotherapy and
eventual control of human cancer.*

Preface

Cancer exacts an incredibly destructive toll on the world's human populations. In recent years we have frequently heard the expression "war on cancer," but compared to the carnage inflicted by cancer, our scientific and medical efforts, to date, would seem more like a minor skirmish.

Some comprehension of the cancer problem can be obtained from a look at the current and projected casualty list for the United States. In this country, about 700,000 new cases of cancer will be diagnosed in 1976 and over 1 million known cases will continue to be treated. Over 400,000 of these patients will die from cancer in our bicentennial year. With the incidence of cancer in the United States increasing to 5.2% in 1975, compared to the 1.1% yearly rate experienced for decades, Dr. F. J. Rauscher, Jr.,[338] Director of the National Cancer Institute, has estimated that more than 10 million people will be under treatment for cancer and nearly 4 million will expire from cancer in this decade. At that rate, cancer will appear in nearly two of three families and the necessary medical care will cost some $15–20 billion per year. Thus unless methods for the treatment and control of cancer are markedly improved, about 53 million Americans now alive will eventually be cancer patients. Unfortunately the major types of human cancer are still beyond curative care by surgical and radiological techniques and because of the paucity of currently available cancer chemotherapeutic drugs with curative potential.

The best hope for future control and curative treatment of cancer depends upon widespread application of preventive measures and the further discovery and development of anti-cancer drugs of both synthetic and biosynthetic origin. Both of the latter approaches to cancer therapy gained increasing support during the 1940's. Now we have reached the stage at which very useful drugs of synthetic and natural origin have been developed, especially in the U.S. National Cancer Institution's programs, capable of curative treatment for 11 types of human cancer.

The search for cancer chemotherapeutic natural products has been rapidly accelerating in recent years and holds promise of leading to spectacular developments in cancer treatment over the next decade. Current clinical successes with actinomycin D, adriamycin, and vincristine (combined with the current potential of other biosynthetic products such as maytansine) have been quite promising. Now the search for still more effective cancer chemotherapeutic agents must receive the vigorous (and increased) support necessary to uncover the even more selective and effective cancer chemotherapy drugs of the future. The same must be said for the increased support urgently needed to explore further the synthetic modification of natural anticancer agents and the exploratory synthesis of cancer chemotherapeutic drugs.

The cancer research program now at Arizona State University was initiated in September 1957 at the University of Maine, and later that fall this writer agreed to undertake an evaluation of the Labiatae plant family for antineoplastic constituents as part of the newly organized National Cancer Institute program of systematic study of plants and microorganisms as sources of cancer chemotherapeutic agents. The first shipments of Labiatae extracts to the National Cancer Institute were made during the following year, but because of severe financial limitations, our plant program remained in barely active form for the next 10 years. Over this period, major emphasis was placed on synthesis of potential antineoplastic agents and synthetic modification of naturally occurring anticancer and cytotoxic substances. However, in 1966, it was possible to initiate substantial efforts in the then-unexplored fields of arthropod and marine animal antineoplastic constituents. By 1969, these endeavors concerned with plant and animal anticancer agents accounted for nearly 90% of our total commitment. In this same period, the 1969 review of plant anticancer agents by Hartwell and Abbott[145] and the 1967 review of naturally occurring anticancer agents by Neuss and colleagues[277] were made available. In the past 5 years, progress concerned with anticancer agents of biosynthetic origin has been rapidly increasing, and the need for a current treatment of the subject led to preparation of this survey.

The principal objective of Volume 1 is to provide a current (to February 1976) overall view of the cancer problem and the development of cancer chemotherapeutic drugs of biosynthetic origin. In addition, it is hoped that the approach employed in Volume 1 will give the chemist and the biologist an appreciation of cancer treatment and the physician a view of how biosynthetic antineoplastic agents are discovered and developed. Volume 2 was prepared to provide a tabular summary (to April 1976) of all the naturally occurring antineoplastic and cytotoxic substances described in the chemical literature. In total, it is hoped that this effort to correlate and bring up to date the chemistry and cancer biology of biosynthetic anticancer agents will prove useful to a variety of disciplines and assist in advancing future progress toward better and more readily available cancer chemotherapeutic drugs with not only curative potential but far-reaching curative action.

Many of the most significant and invaluable advances in the field of biosynthetic cancer chemotherapeutic agents witnessed, particularly over the past 10 years, are due in large measure to a number of scientists and clinicians at the National Cancer Institute whose brilliant leadership and devotion to duty has inspired and promoted this progress. Here I would like to single out for special recognition in cancer chemotherapeutic drug development Drs. John D. Douros, Robert R. Engle, Jonathan L. Hartwell, Ronald B. Ross, Harry B. Wood, and C. Gordon Zubrod. Other most admirable contributions have been made to the biological and clinical aspects of the NCI drug development program by, for example, Miss B. J. Abbott and Drs. P. P. Carbone, S. K. Carter, V. T. DeVita, A. Goldin, V. T. Oliverio, J. M. Venditti, and M. D. Walker. In respect to this work, I am very pleased to acknowledge the expert and splendid contributions of Mrs. Christine H. Duplissa and Mrs. Marie D. Baughman in final preparation of the manuscript.

George R. Pettit.

Paradise Valley, Arizona

Contents

"Accuse not Nature, she hath done her part;
Do thou but thine!"

Milton—*Paradise Lost*

Chapter 1

Introduction and Perspective

Cancer is the general term for a series of neoplastic (*Gr. neos* new, *plasma* formation) diseases that are characterized by changes in a cell leading to abnormal (unordered and uncontrolled) cellular proliferation. Cancer is commonly encountered in all animals except the lower forms (see Chapter 9), and even plants develop growths that resemble cancer. Cancer is well known in all human populations and has probably been with us from the beginning of time. Indeed some fossilized dinosaur bones have been located that seem to reflect damage attributable to cancer.

In the broadest sense, neoplastic disease can be divided into benign and malignant categories. A benign tumor is generally contained within a membrane of connective tissue, and histologically all cells appear alike and derived from one tissue source. Unlike malignant tumors, they do not metastasize. At the start, malignant tumor cells may maintain some degree of their original specialized function, structure, and relationship to the tissue cells of origin. By maintaining this degree of differentiation, some cancer cells can at an early stage still perform some limited useful activity. However, as the disease progresses, the histological changes become more apparent until the cell is no longer recognizable. At this point dramatic structural and functional changes are obvious.

The uncontrolled cellular advance characteristic of malignant neoplastic disease does not necessarily mean a more rapid rate of cell growth, since cancer cells have the same variations in growth rates as do normal cells. However, if this process is not arrested, it will progress to cause death. The usual relentless progression of human cancer is due to the tendency toward metastases as malignant cells leave the original site and circulate in the blood and lymph systems to initiate abnormal growth at other sites in the body. Metastases may not occur until the primary site has reached an easily detectable size. The time interval for metastases may range from a very short period to many years. In this period, metastases may form by the hundreds in widely separated parts of the body. Usually these metastases proceed by way of the lymph system, and regional lymph nodes are frequently the first points of attack. In many cases, the actual route of metastases can be predicted and, in the more common types of cancer, is well known. For example, in breast cancer, metastases to the thoracic cavity, lungs, liver, and bones are frequently seen, and in lung cancer metastases to the liver, brain, adrenals, and bone are the common routes. Interestingly some types of tissue are less attractive for metastases; these include the spleen, the heart, the kidney, the prostate, the thyroid, the breast, and skeletal muscle.

Biological classification of cancer is based on both the type of cell and tissue involved.[272] The majority of human cancer is of the carcinoma type, that is, solid tumors derived from epithelial tissues. These comprise the internal and external surfaces of the body as well as the colon and derived organs, which include the mucus membranes, the skin, the pancreas, the thyroid, the prostate, the liver, and the breast. The human carcinomas comprise about 95% of all malignancies. The next 3–4% of human cancer is made up of tumors affecting mixed tissues, such as the testes and the ovaries. The remaining percentage (about 2%) of human cancer is of the sarcoma type. The sarcomas are solid tumors derived from embryonal mesoderm and thus arise in connective tissues, such as cartilage, muscle, fibrous connective tissue, and bone. Sarcomas are very prominent among the experimental animals usually employed for studies in the cancer field. The gliomas and the other tumors of the central nervous system are usually given separate classification. Varieties of cancer that are both carcinomas and sarcomas are designated carcinosarcoma. Another commonly-referred-to cancer classification is that of melanoma, which has its start in the melanocytes, or pigment-synthesizing cells, such as in the skin, the eyes, and the meninges. Malignant melanoma[63] usually metastasizes into regional lymph nodes, the liver, the lungs, and the brain. And melanocarcinoma even metastasizes to the heart. Approximately 90% of melanoma begins in the skin and most of the remainder in the eye. In 1975, preparation of a cell line from a patient with malignant melanoma was reported[112] and may prove useful for anticancer drug evaluation. Although melanoma constitutes about 2% of human cancer, it occurs throughout the world's population in all age groups and in both sexes.

The leukemias and lymphomas are considered systematic diseases and are given separate classification. Hematological malignancies of the leukemic variety affect the blood-forming tissues—that is, the bone marrow, the lymph nodes, and the reticuloendothelial system—and usually lead to abnormal production of leukocytes (commonly known as white blood cells) by the bone marrow. However, most of these leukocytes do not become the type useful in fending off infection. Instead defenses against infection are reduced, and the leukemic cells become disseminated throughout the blood and lymph systems, where they continue to proliferate. In the acute forms and in later stages of chronic leukemia, the malignant cells spread beyond the blood-forming tissues. Generally, when the cells are poorly differentiated, the rapid onset typical of acute leukemia is experienced. The common leukemias are classed as lymphocytic (malignant lymphocytes), granulocytic or myelocytic (characteristic granules in the leukocyte cytoplasm), monocytic (leukocytes with horeshoe-shaped nuclei), and stem-cell (primitive malignant leukocytes).

The lymphomas are used to characterize a series of neoplastic diseases of varying malignancy that begin in the bone marrow, the lymph nodes, the spleen, or the thymus and result in the production of abnormal numbers of lymphocytes. The lymphomas migrate among the lymphoid tissues and, in advanced stages, implicate surrounding tissues and the central nervous system.[238] Hodgkin's disease is a well-known lymphoma characterized by two types of lymph cells. Others include lymphoblastomas (immature lymph cells), lymphocytomas (mature lymph cells), and lymphosarcomas (beginning in lymph nodes or mucosa lymphatic areas). A very useful review of non-Hodgkin lymphomas has been prepared by Jones.[177] In the United States, the leukemias account for 3–4% and the lymphomas some 5–6% of all diagnosed malignancies.

The metastases that result from the various types of cancer amount to multiple attacks throughout the body that then interfere with normal organ processes and lead to the fatal result in a majority of patients. Contrary to popular belief, the neoplastic disease is not usually the direct cause of death; instead the patient is more likely to expire from the result of biological damage caused by the cancer, ranging from the bleeding, perforation, or obstruction resulting from colon cancer to infection or emaciation (cachexia). A recent analysis[167] of the more than 500 deaths per year due to cancer at the M. D. Anderson Hospital and Tumor Institute provides a good illustration of this point. The majority (47%) of the deaths were caused by gram-negative bacilli, primarily *Escherichia coli, Pseudomonas* spp., and *Klebsiella* spp., leading to pneumonia, peritonitis, or septicemia. Organ failure accounted for 25%, infarction 11%, carcinomatosis 10%, and hemorrhage 7%. Fortunately the survival rates of patients with cancer should now be on the increase because of a combination of early diagnosis, increasing application of cancer chemotherapy, and improvements in supportive, surgical, and radiological techniques and in endocrine therapy.[71] Here it must be emphasized that each type of human cancer has a definite set of symptoms and requires a specific course of treatment. Ideally the best course of treatment would be at the outset of hyperplasia and would involve containment or reversal.

There is overwhelming evidence that a majority of human cancers can be attributed to one or more of the following means of biological insult, acting singly or in combination: radiation (X-rays, solar, ultraviolet, ionizing, from nuclear fission, radioactive particles of tobacco smoke,[255] radium, radon, and uranium), carcinogens [asbestos, benzene, aromatic hydrocarbons from coal tar, creosote, cutting oils, pitch, tobacco smoke and soot, aromatic amines such as α-naphthyl amine, N-nitrosoamines, some bis(2-chloroethyl)-amines, diethylstilbesterol, arsenic compounds and chromates, and fungal and other plant products, as well as betel-nut and tobacco chewing], trauma (injury with continual irritation), and viruses. Occupational exposure, especially to asbestos, for example, of the chrysotile $(Mg_3Si_2O_5(OH)_4)$ type can lead to exceedingly high risk of developing carcinoma and mesothelioma of the lungs, the pleura, and the peritoneum.[126] Of course every reasonable means should be taken to prevent employment contact with carcinogenic industrial chemicals and to protect the public from various carcinogens (such as the pesticides chlordan and heptachlor) carried into our environment as air and water pollutants and/or food contaminants. By way of illustration, aflatoxin B_1 (**1**, one of a series of closely related, highly carcinogenic constituents of the fungus *Aspergillus*) and other such carcinogenic fungal metabolites are now of great concern to the food industry, and efforts are being made to eliminate potentially hazardous materials, such as moldy peanuts.[20,132] The decreasing incidence of stomach cancer in the United States might be related to the decreasing use of moldy foods, and the higher incidence of liver cancer, for example, in China[299] might be due to the consumption of such moldy foods. Several other plant products have been strongly implicated in human cancer. Cycasin (**2**, a constituent of the African cycad nut), safrole (**3**, a sassafras oil constituent that was formerly used in root beer), and the Senecio alkaloid lasiocarpine (**4**, a component of certain herbal medicines) are well-established human carcinogens. The N-nitrosoamines arising from sodium nitrite used to preserve various meat products (hot dogs, etc.) and from other sources in

1

Aflatoxin B$_1$

2

Cycasin

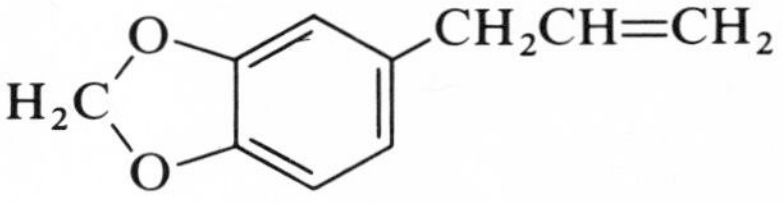

3

Safrole

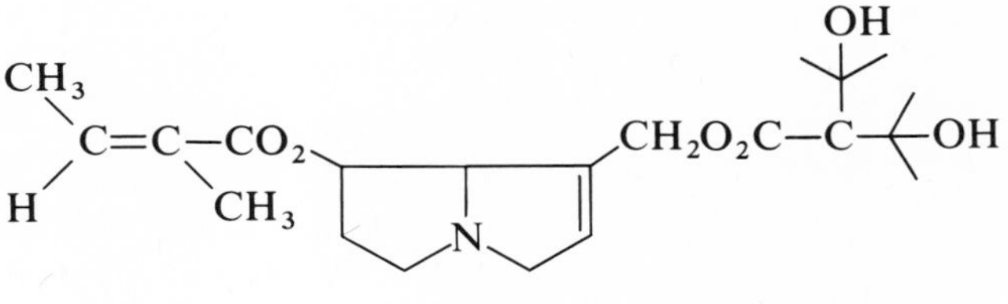

4

Lasiocarpine

the diet represent a most serious cancer hazard. In addition, coffee and other phenolic foodstuffs may catalyze *N*-nitrosoamine formation in the digestive tract.[56]

The general population is also exposed to many hazards of a lesser known and more insidious nature, which include the great variety of food colors (especially Red Dyes No. 2 and No. 4 and Carbon Black, which have just been banned by the FDA as possible human carcinogens),[419,420] flavorings, and preservatives added to food, as well as to various cosmetics and other such proprietary items.

Other factors known to play prominent roles in human cancer range from dietary intake[94a] (high beef and fat intake, combined with low roughage, may be related to colon cancer, and a high caloric intake may be related to other types)[436] to cancer resulting from implanted plastic products and proximity to chemical and other industrial plants.[164] Indeed ingredients of the daily diet may cause, directly or indirectly, 50% of all cancer in American women and 30% of all cancer in American men.[39]

In the United States, the most obvious and well-defined carcinogen sources in dire need of preventive measures are the heavy consumption and use of tobacco and alcohol.[94a] In addition to lung cancer,[364] tobacco smoking has also been related to cancer of the oral cavity, the larynx, the esophagus, and the bladder. Deaths of many other types related to tobacco smoking, such as myocardial infarction,[431] are well known. Similarly alcoholism has been related to cancer of the oral cavity, the larynx, the esophagus, the liver, and possibly the pancreas.[78] Incidence of the latter neoplastic disease is increasing rapidly in the United States, and the rate of increase is now second only to that of lung cancer. Pancreatic carcinoma currently ranks fourth among cancer deaths in the United States; the current dismal treatment picture has been analyzed by Carter and Comis.[52] Unfortunately between the very addictive[286,352] nature of both tobacco smoke and alcohol and the excellent business they provide (603 *billion* cigarettes sold in the United States in 1975, up from 594.5 billion in 1974 and 547.2 billion in 1971), reduction and/or elimination of these causes of cancer present great challenges. This sorry fact has been emphasized by

Shimkin[371] and many others. Elimination or reduction in personal use of both tobacco and alcohol in the United States would remove at least two-thirds of lung cancer deaths and at least half of cancer deaths originating in the oral cavity, the larynx, and the esophagus. Unless the distribution of marijuana can be effectively controlled (or better eliminated), cancer from this type of smoking will become an even more serious problem. Marijuana cigarettes have been shown to produce higher concentrations of carcinogens than those made from tobacco.[285] In this respect, Ochsner[286] has referred to a quote by deMontaigne, who observed in the 16th century, "Men do not usually die, they kill themselves."

Of course, a rapidly growing list of other substances ranging from chlorinated hydrocarbons to the pyridine derivative isoniazid (**5**) and the amino acid ethionine (**6**) have been shown to induce cancer rapidly in experimental animals. No doubt many of these same compounds, such as chloroform and chlordan, hold great hazards for man. The recent discovery of the relationship between the exposure of vinyl plastic workers to vinyl chloride and their development of angiosarcoma is now well known and provides ample illustration.

The human cancer resulting from exposure to chemical carcinogens was first observed among chimney sweeps 200 years ago in England and has been reviewed by Weisburger.[427] A number of interesting theories have been proposed to explain such carcinogenic activity,[98,427] and a current hypothesis for certain carcinogenic hydrocarbons provides an illustration. The Pullmans[331] have suggested that the carcinogenic activity of some aromatic hydrocarbons depends on a region of high olefinic character (K region)[14a] with the remainder (L region) of low olefinic character and reactivity. Then enzymatic oxidation of the K bond to an epoxide would yield an intermediate capable of reaction with proteins and nucleic acids.[437] Calvin[45] has recently discussed another carcinogenesis proposal.

Over the past nearly 70 years, more than 120 viruses have been characterized that induce tumors in lower animals. These viruses are capable of initiating in a wide variety of vertebrates cancers that resemble most of the human types of cancer. A

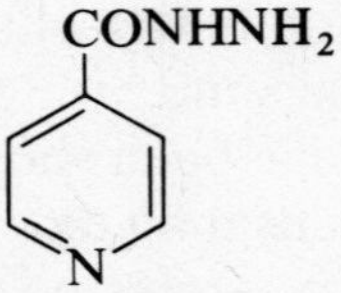

$$CONHNH_2$$

5

Isoniazid

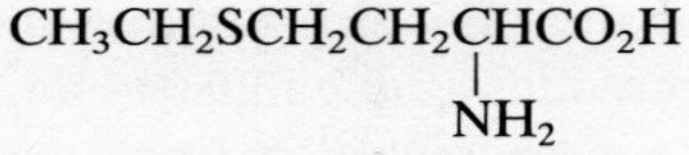

$$CH_3CH_2SCH_2CH_2CHCO_2H$$
$$NH_2$$

6

Ethionine

series of authoritative reviews of this subject have recently been prepared.[22,60,339] Rauscher and O'Connor[339] have also reviewed the possibility that cells already contain endogenous virogenes (genetic material that encodes information for the production of complete viruses) and oncogenes (which encode information for the production of substances that will produce neoplastic transformation) and that these potentially lethal chemical transformations can be triggered (derepression) by radiation, chemical carcinogens, viruses, genetic defects, mutant genes, and eventually the aging process. Another statement of this hypothesis has recently been made by Temin.[395] While this theory is very attractive as a unified concept, it should in no way dampen enthusiasm for discovering cancer chemotherapeutic agents for cancer treatment and cure. Substances can certainly be discovered that will repress any endogenous oncogene(s) and stimulate the human immunological system to greater effectiveness.

Of the vertebrate groups studied, each either carries its own oncogenic viruses or is a suitable host for inoculation of those from other species. When the same experimental methods are applied to human cancer, three categories of virus or viruslike particles have been detected and/or isolated. Morphologically similar RNA[267] viruses of the B type have been found in tissue culture lines derived from human breast cancer and in the milk of women from families with a high rate of breast cancer, including normal women of the inbred Parsi sect of Bombay, which has a high incidence of breast cancer. By means of thin-section electron microscopy, oncogenic RNA viruses have been detected in approximately 3% of milk specimens from normal women and 25% from former breast cancer patients where one breast has been surgically removed.[59]

Here it should be mentioned that some oncogenic viruses are not visible by electron microscopy because they have become incorporated into the cellular genetic components. A general method of locating viruses in cellular material is to detect the corresponding viral antibody produced by the host through immunofluorescence techniques (tagging with a fluorescent dye and visualization by ultraviolet light). A new approach is based on the fact that an enzyme common to all oncogenic viruses in animals so far studied and believed absent in other types of viruses can now be utilized. This enzyme is responsible for an RNA-to-DNA information transfer and has been designated an RNA-dependent DNA polymerase or reverse transcriptase as reported in 1970 by Temin and Mitutani[396] and Baltimore.[17] The potential for biosynthetic interference with the normal function of this oncogenic enzyme opens another vista for biosynthetic or synthetic drug controls.

The herpes-type viruses related to those that cause fever blisters and infectious mononucleosis have been detected by electron microscopy in various human cancer tissue cultures including blood samples from patients with chronic leukemia. While infectious mononucleosis is nonmalignant, it does involve cells of the same type involved in leukemia. Such cells rapidly proliferate and for a short time appear as if malignant. One of the herpes-type viruses believed to be oncogenic is the Epstein–Barr virus known as EBV. A compelling summary of the evidence implicating EBV as oncogenic for man has been summarized by Rauscher and O'Connor.[339] One of the most striking facts is that EBV and/or high levels of antibody to the virus are detectable in all patients with carcinoma of the nasopharynx and with Burkitt's lymphoma (in Africa). Thus EBV, like infectious mononucleosis, seems to be transmitted horizontally, and a vaccine approach to prevention seems feasible.

The C-type viruses with characteristic double encapsulating membranes were first studied in murine leukemia some 40 years ago. Subsequently the C-type viruses have been found capable of inducing both leukemia and sarcomas in a variety of birds and mammals. More specifically, the C-type RNA viruses are responsible for lymphomas and sarcomas in, for example, cats, chickens, hamsters, and mice. Also the herpeslike viruses are known to cause adenocarcinomas in frogs and lymphomas in monkeys.

Very importantly, Hodgkin's disease, on the basis of epidemiological studies,[410] seems to have an infectious etiology. While herpeslike viruses seem to be eliminated in the case of Hodgkin's disease, there is very interesting circumstantial evidence implicating the C-type viruses.[160] In the plasma of patients with Hodgkin's disease, a 31% incidence of C-type virus particles was detected. This compares with a 14% prevalence in various types of acute leukemia and a 43% rate in acute myelogenous leukemia. However, De Vita and colleagues[160] have emphasized that the C-type particles they located did not exhibit budding from the cells of malignant tissues, which is very characteristic of C-type viruses. Furthermore by thin-section electron microscopy, it was not possible to eliminate completely the possibility that these particles were some sort of membrane remnant. Tissue lines from human lymphomas and sarcomas may in the future give more definitive results.

The C-type viruses are quite complex and appear to be composed of eight or more proteins,[380] a high lipid concentration, and only a small amount of nucleic acid (1–2%). They have the property of being able to elicit both type-specific and group-specific antigens. The type C viruses may be responsible for human sarcomas and have definitely been linked to human leukemia. The sarcoma evidence is based on antigenic studies, but continuous production of budding type C viruses from a patient with acute myelogenous leukemia has just been achieved by Gallagher and Gallo.[106,267] Successful isolation of the type C virus was made possible by discovery of a factor released by certain growing cells that is capable of supporting the exponential growth of leukemic myeloid leukocytes. Interestingly the patient, a 61-year-old woman, had no prior family history of leukemia or lymphoma but did have contact with a friend with leukemia prior to the rapid onset of her neoplastic disease. The excellent advance made by Gallo and colleagues further increases the prospects for eventually developing a vaccine for hematological malignancies and sarcomas. However, very formidable practical and ethical difficulties stand in the way of developing and proving the effectiveness of human cancer vaccines.

While the necessary knowledge has already been developed for preventing a very large number of eventual cancer deaths and needs only to be implemented, the necessary knowledge for curative treatment and overall control is still at an early though promising stage. On a short-term basis, the objective of cancer treatment research is to extend the period of disease-free remission and increase the number of patients responding to treatment and for the long term to develop methods for the cure and complete control of human cancer. The term *cancer cure* has been defined by Zubrod[442] and is applied to those patients with clinically proven cancer that, following treatment, should have a normal life expectancy as compared with the predicted survival of all people in our population of the same sex and age.

In most cases, chances for curative cancer treatment are best when cancer is first diagnosed, and there is now ample clinical evidence that a combination of treatment methods designed to have a maximum effect on a specific type of neoplastic disease produces the highest survival and cure rates. Currently about one-third of all cancer patients can be cured, and this achievement might be raised to one-half if each patient had the best care and treatment available. Indeed most cancer patients have the best chances for extended survival or cure if they are first treated by an experienced team of physicians in a medical center with the resources necessary to apply all forms of effective therapy.

In the past, surgery and/or X-irradiation have been the most commonly used modalities for cancer treatment. But both are capable of curing only truly localized cancer.[441] However, at the time of diagnosis, the situation is usually one of metastatic cancer that has already spread to distant tissue sites. In such cases, Zubrod[443] and Perry[296] have estimated that with the best diagnostic techniques, one cannot detect an internal tumor unless it already contains at least 1 billion cells and is in a suitable location. However, most internal solid tumors as well as the leukemias and lymphomas do not become readily diagnosible until the neoplastic cell concentration numbers some $1 \times$

10^{12}. As an example, it is possible to detect a 1-cm malignant lesion in the lung and remove it surgically, but it is well known that the present cure rate for lung cancer is dismally low and ranges from a very low percentage with some types to 14% overall for respiratory cancer.

As just noted, a patient with barely detectable cancer at the time of diagnosis may already have 10^{12} cancer cells, which has led the well-known oncology surgeon Rhoads to remark that "the pervasive persistence of the underlying concept that the main value of surgical therapy in cancer lies in total excision of a localized cancer can no longer be believed because it is not supported by experience but this lays upon us the responsibility of finding out how it helps and of redefining our indications."[344] Probably the same observation can be applied to much of radiotherapy as currently employed. In the past, radiotherapy has been most frequently used as a palliative, for example, to relieve the pain in inoperable cancer of the colon and liver.[379] The curative potential of radiotherapy has probably been best illustrated in the case of Hodgkin's disease by Rosenberg and Kaplan.[349]

Unfortunately each of the major treatment modalities for cancer has serious limitations. The cosmetic and anatomical deficiencies arising from surgical procedures are well known and range from simple amputation to the profound trauma of facial loss. Furthermore there is now ample evidence against the use of radical surgical procedures, especially with breast cancer, bronchial cancer, rectal cancer (electrocoagulation of rectal cancer is superior to the usual rectal abdominoperineal excision), and stomach cancer (no gain in total compared to subtotal gastrectomy; life is much better for the patient with a subtotal procedure).[114] Even worse is the growing evidence that a major surgical operation can depress the patient's immune mechanism against cancer![114,77]

The side effects of irradiation are not always immediately evident but can also be severe and nonreversible.[441] Such side effects include risk of massive hemorrhage,[94b] permanent bone or muscle atrophy, severe mental defects, unsightly skin lesions, cardiopulmonary failure, and the insidious long-term genetic and carcinogenic effects.[377a] With chemotherapy, most of the serious side effects are quickly reversible once the drug treatment has ceased. Such toxic reactions are usually found in the bone marrow, the hair roots, the lymph nodes, and the gastrointestinal epithelium. These sites have a high growth fraction undergoing DNA synthesis. An explanation of the latter concept is provided later on in this chapter. A variety of other toxic side effects have been noted that involve the bladder, the central nervous system, the heart, the liver, the lung, the kidney, and the pancreas, but most are reversible.[443] Fortunately good cancer chemotherapeutic drugs can be distributed throughout the patient's body and destroy neoplastic cells that are otherwise unreachable by surgical and/or radiotherapy techniques. Therefore the best current treatment approach would seem to be early and extensive application of anticancer drugs to control undetected metastatic cancer and limited (reasonable) surgery and/or irradiation to control localized neoplastic disease.

Organized cancer chemotherapy and treatment programs are conducted principally in the United States, the Soviet Union, the People's Republic of China, Japan, and Europe (under the auspices of the European Organization for Research on Treatment of Cancer).[50] In the United States, the National Cancer Institute has been leading the attack on the cancer problem and has been exploring appropriate and effective combinations of various treatment modalities. These approaches are primarily chemotherapy, surgery, radiation, supportive therapy (antibiotics and protective isolation), and immunotherapy. In the latter area, attempts are being made to increase the immune responses of patients with advanced neoplastic disease.[274] Experimentally, immunity to certain animal cancer has been demonstrated by treatment of the lymphoid cells of a nonimmune animal with the RNA from its immune counterpart. Also some patients with acute leukemia or melanoma have benefited through stimulation of their immune reactions with the attenuated tuberculosis bacillus BCG. Morton and co-workers[163] have found intralesional injection with BCG vaccine to be the best treatment for patients with intradermal transient metastases from malignant melanoma and for selected patients with local recurrence of breast cancer. They have also found 2,4-dinitrochlorobenzene a very satisfactory topical treatment for some patients with basal- or squamous-cell carcinoma. Perhaps some of the better anticancer drugs also act in part by stimulating a suitable immune response in the patient. Eventual progress in immunotherapy may provide a means for eradicating neoplastic cells missed by chemotherapy. Now it would seem that whenever feasible, the major mass of cancer cells should be removed by surgery with concomitant cancer chemotherapy to control metastatic cancer and reduce the number of neoplastic cells to the point where the patient's own immune system can again function properly. Eventually, when a greater number of more effective and curative cancer chemotherapeutic drugs have been developed, it should be possible to avoid the more debilitating surgical and radiological procedures now in general use.

In the National Cancer Institute's Division of Cancer Treatment, antineoplastic drugs have already been developed that produce normal life expectancy in patients with acute lymphocytic leukemia, Burkitt's lymphoma, choriocarcinoma, embryonal testicular tumors, Ewing's sarcoma, Hodgkin's disease, non-Hodgkin's lymphomas, mycosis fungoides, retinoblastoma, rabdomyosarcoma, and Wilms' tumor. Osteogenic sarcoma should soon become the next addition to this most stimulating list. For certain of these neoplastic diseases, such as Burkitt's lymphoma and choriocarcinoma, cures are achieved with just one drug (methotrexate or cytoxan) treatment. With others, such as Hodgkin's disease, a four-drug combination is required, and with several, the anticancer drug is a necessary part of surgery and/or radiation treatment to effect cures. These recent successful treatment methods range from approximate cure rates of 20% with metastatic embryonal testicular cancer to 75% for choriocarcinoma and nearly 90% for patients with Wilms' tumor. Similarly the curative (52%, 5-year survival rate) chemotherapeutic treatment for Ewing's sarcoma developed by the National Cancer Institute has been improved recently through the use of alternating high-dose applications of adriamycin and cytoxan-vincristine.[328]

To date, about 50 synthetic and biosynthetic (including hormones) compounds have been found of use in the clinical management of cancer. Of these, 36 are now available commercially, and 25 as single agents are capable of causing regression of certain human neoplastic diseases. A valuable summary covering 32 of the drugs useful in cancer treatment has been prepared by Carter,[53] who has kindly allowed the use of this information for reference in Table 1. Further clinical study of these drugs (and others such as those represented by structures **8**, **11**, **12**, **13**, **15**, **19**, **20**, and **28**) and of newer, potentially more effective ones currently under development in the National Cancer Institute's programs offers exciting prospects for further advances in direct and adjuvant chemotherapy. The utility of cancer chemotherapy to eradicate the microscopic segments of a neoplastic disease has been demonstrated many times and is well established in the areas of Hodgkin's disease, Ewing's sarcoma, osteogenic sarcoma, and Wilms' tumor. An instructive account of recent progress in cancer chemotherapy has been prepared by Zubrod,[442,444] who led the NCI cancer chemotherapy program responsible for many of these recent advances.

Two recent conquests by cancer chemotherapy serve to illustrate the potential of this approach to the control and cure of disseminated cancer of both the hematological and the solid types. The development of the four-drug treatment known as *MOPP* at the National Cancer Institute by De Vita and colleagues[80] has caused a most beneficial revolution in the treatment of Hodgkin's disease and has recently led to a significant increase in survival time in oat cell carcinoma of the lung.[281a] The best treatment protocol for advanced Hodgkin's disease is six courses at monthly intervals of the mustargen (cytoxan), oncovin (vincristine), procarbazine, and prednisone combination. In the original study, 81% of the patients achieved complete remission, and including those achieving partial remission,

Table 1. *Commercially Available Cancer Chemotherapeutic Drugs*

Drug	Usual dosage	Toxicity		Major indications
		Acute	Delayed	
Alkylating Agents:				
Busulfan (Myleran) (26)	2–8 mg/day for 2–3 wks PO; stop for recovery; then maintenance	None	Bone marrow depression	Chronic granulocytic leukemia
Chlorambucil (Leukeran) (9)	Start 0.1–0.2 mg/kg/day PO; adjust for maintenance	None	Bone marrow depression (anemia, leukopenia, and thrombocytopenia) can be severe with excessive dosage	Chronic lymphocytic leukemia, Hodgkin's disease, non-Hodgkin's lymphoma, trophoblastic neoplasms
Cyclophosphamide (Cytoxan) (7)	40 mg/kg IV in single or in 2–8 daily doses or 2–4 mg/kg/day PO for 10 days; adjust for maintenance	Nausea and vomiting	Bone marrow depression, alopecia, cystitis	Hodgkin's disease and other lymphomas, multiple myeloma, lymphocytic leukemia, many solid cancers
Mechlorethamine (nitrogen mustard; HN$_2$, Mustargen) (10)	0.4 mg/kg IV in single or divided doses	Nausea and vomiting	Moderate depression of peripheral blood count	Hodgkin's disease and other lymphomas, bronchogenic carcinoma
Melphalan (1-phenylala-nine mustard; Alkeran) (14)	0.25 mg/kg/day for 4 days PO; 2–4 mg/day as maintenance or 0.1–0.15 mg/kg/day for 2–3 wks	None	Bone marrow depression	Multiple myeloma, malignant melanoma, ovarian carcinoma, testicular seminoma

(Table 1 continued)

Table 1—continued

Drug	Usual dosage	Toxicity		Major indications
		Acute	Delayed	
Thiotepa (triethylene-thiophosphoramide) (16)	0.2 mg/kg IV for 5 days	None	Bone marrow depression	Hodgkin's disease, bronchogenic and breast carcinomas
Antimetabolites: Cytarabine hydrochloride (arabinosyl cytosine; Cytosar) (17)	2–3 mg/kg/day IV until response or toxicity or 1–3 mg/kg IV over 24 hours for up to 10 days	Nausea and vomiting	Bone marrow depression, megaloblastosis	Acute leukemia
Fluorouracil (5-FU, FU) (18)	12.5 mg/kg/day IV for 3–5 days or 15 mg/kg/wk for 6 wks	Nausea	Oral and gastrointestinal ulceration, stomatitis and diarrhea, bone marrow depression	Breast, large bowel, and ovarian cancer
Mercaptopurine (6-MP, Purinethol) (21)	2.5 mg/kg/day PO	Occasional nausea and vomiting, usually well tolerated	Bone marrow depression, occasional hepatic damage	Acute lymphocytic and granulocytic leukemia, chronic granulocytic leukemia
Methotrexate (amethopterin; MTX) (22)	2.5–5.0 mg/day PO; 0.4 mg/kg rapid IV daily 4–5 days (not over 25 mg) or 0.4 mg/kg rapid IV twice/wk	Occasional diarrhea, hepatic necrosis	Oral and gastrointestinal ulceration, bone marrow depression (anemia, leukopenia, thrombocytopenia), cirrhosis	Acute lymphocytic leukemia, choriocarcinoma, carcinoma of cervix and head and neck area, mycosis fungoides, solid cancers

Drug	Dose	Acute toxicity	Delayed toxicity	Indications
Thioguanine (6-TG) (23)	2 mg/kg/day PO	Occasional nausea and vomiting, usually well tolerated	Bone marrow depression	Acute leukemia
Plant Alkaloids				
Vinblastine sulfate (Velban) (105)	0.1–0.2 mg/kg/wk IV or q 2 wks	Nausea and vomiting, local irritant	Alopecia, stomatitis, bone marrow depression, loss of reflexes	Hodgkin's disease and other lymphomas, solid cancers
Vincristine sulfate (Oncovin) (104)	0.01–0.03 mg/kg/wk IV	Local irritant	Areflexia, peripheral neuritis, paralytic ileus, mild bone marrow depression	Acute lymphocytic leukemia, Hodgkin's disease and other lymphomas, solid cancers
Antibiotics				
Adriamycin (Doxorubicin) (136)	60–90 mg/m² IV, single dose or over 3 days; repeat q 3 wks to total dose 550 mg/m²	Nausea, red urine (not hematuria)	Bone marrow depression, cardiotoxicity, alopecia, stomatitis	Soft tissue, osteogenic and miscellaneous sarcomas, Hodgkin's disease, non-Hodgkin's lymphoma, bronchogenic and breast carcinoma, thyroid cancer
Bleomycin (Blenoxane) (145)	10–15 mg/m²/wk or twice/wk, IV or IM to total dose 300–400 mg	Nausea and vomiting, fever, very toxic	Edema of hands, pulmonary fibrosis, stomatitis, alopecia	Hodgkin's disease, non-Hodgkin's lymphoma, squamous-cell carcinoma (head and neck), testicular carcinoma
Dactinomycin (actinomycin D; Cosmegen) (144)	0.015–0.05 mg/kg/wk (1–2.5 mg) 3–5 wks IV; wait for marrow recovery (3–4 wks) then repeat course	Nausea and vomiting, local irritant	Stomatitis, oral ulcers, diarrhea, alopecia, mental depression, bone marrow depression	Testicular carcinoma, Wilms' tumor, rhabdomyosarcoma, Ewing's and osteogenic sarcoma, and other solid tumors

(Table 1 continued)

Table 1—continued

		Toxicity		
Drug	Usual dosage	Acute	Delayed	Major indications
Mithramycin (Mithracin) (132)	0.025–0.050 mg/kg q 2 days for up to 8 doses, IV	Nausea and vomiting, hepatotoxicity	Bone marrow depression (thrombocytopenia), hypocalcemia	Testicular carcinoma, trophoblastic neoplasms
Mitomycin C (Mutamycin) (129)	0.05 mg/kg/day IV for 5 days	Nausea and vomiting, "flulike syndrome"	Bone marrow depression, skin toxicity; pulmonary, renal, CNS effects	Squamous-cell carcinoma of head and neck, lungs and cervix; adenocarcinoma of the stomach, pancreas, colon, rectum; adeno- and duct-cell carcinoma of the breast
Other Synthetic Agents				
Dacarbazine (DTIC-Dome; DIC) (24)	4.5 mg/kg/day IV for 10 days; repeated q 28 days	Nausea and vomiting "flulike syndrome"	Bone marrow depression (rare)	Metastatic malignant melanoma
Hydroxyurea (Hydrea) (25)	80 mg/kg PO single dose q 3 days or 20–30 mg/kg/day PO	Mild nausea and vomiting	Bone marrow depression	Chronic granulocytic leukemia
Mitotane (ortho para DDD o,p′ DDD; Lysodren) (25a)	6–15 mg/kg/day PO	Nausea and vomiting	Dermatitis, diarrhea, mental depression	Adrenal cortical carcinoma

Procarbazine hydrochloride (Methyl hydrazine; ibenzmethyzin; Matulane) (27)	Start 1–2 mg/kg/day PO; increase over 1 wk to 3 mg/kg; maintain for 3 wks then reduce to 2 mg/kg/day until toxicity	Nausea and vomiting	Bone marrow depression CNS depression	Hodgkin's disease, lymphoma, bronchogenic carcinoma
Hormones				
Diethylstilbestrol (DES) (29)	15 mg/day PO (1 mg in prostate cancer)	None	Fluid retention, hypercalcemia, feminization, uterine bleeding; if during pregnancy, may cause vaginal carcinoma in offspring	Breast and prostate carcinomas
Dromostanolone propionate (Drolban) (30)	100 mg 3x/wk, IM	None	Fluid retention, masculinization, hypercalcemia	Breast carcinoma
Ethinyl estradiol (31)	3 mg/day PO	None	Fluid retention, hypercalcemia, feminization, uterine bleeding	Breast and prostate carcinomas
Fluoxymesterone (32)	10–20 mg/day PO	None	Fluid retention, masculinization, cholestatic jaundice	Breast carcinoma
Hydroxyprogesterone caproate (33)	1 Gm IM twice/wk	None	None	Endometrial carcinoma
Medroxyprogesterone acetate (34)	100–200 mg/day PO; 200–600 mg twice/wk	None	None	Endometrial carcinoma, renal-cell, breast cancer

(Table 1 continued)

Table 1—continued

Drug	Usual dosage	Toxicity		Major indications
		Acute	Delayed	
Prednisone (35)	10–100 mg/day PO	None	Hyperadrenocorticism	Acute and chronic lymphocytic leukemia, Hodgkin's disease, non-Hodgkin's lymphomas
Testolactone (Teslac) (36)	100 mg 3x/wk, IM	None	Fluid retention, masculinization	Breast carcinoma
Testosterone enanthate (38)	600–1200 mg/wk, IM	None	Fluid retention, masculinization	Breast carcinoma
Testosterone propionate (37)	50–100 mg, IM 3x/wk	None	Fluid retention, masculinization	Breast carcinoma

the total response rate was 95%. Disease-free survival for 43% of the complete responders has exceeded 5 years, and they are considered cures. To date, this combination chemotherapy has consistently produced a complete response rate of 60–95% and an immediate duration of disease-free survival of over 3 years, and presumably nearly 50% of the complete responders can be considered cured.[119] Interestingly in a new study involving the deletion of prednisone from the MOPP therapy, the complete remission rate dropped to 44%.[37] Generally the MOPP therapy is most effective with patients who have not had prior treatment with extensive irradiation or other types of chemotherapy.[119,349] A very competitive four-drug treatment for Hodgkin's was reported in 1975 by Bonadonna and co-workers.[34] In this approach, a combination (ABVD) of adriamycin, bleomycin, vinblastine, and imidazole carboxamide was employed in a study parallel with that on the use of MOPP. The clinical investigation led by Bonadonna resulted in complete remission in 76% of the Hodgkin's patients treated with MOPP as compared to 75% of those given ABVD. Hopefully this combination will prove useful with patients not responding to MOPP and/or as a method for sequential combination. Also, eliminating the requirement for cyclophosphamide should be very constructive for the future. Recently each of five patients receiving large oral doses (114–295 g over 3–5 years) of cyclophosphamide developed urinary–bladder tumors fatal to four of the five.[418] These patients were being given long-term treatment with very large amounts of cyclophosphamide for various other types of cancer.

The current prospects for combination chemotherapy have been set forth by De Vita.[81] His statement—"now that the chemotherapeutic tools are sharpened, their use in combinations with other modalities in the previously unfamiliar setting of the patient with early stages of the disease promises to lead to an even more exciting chapter in clinical cancer research in the next decade"—reflects the very rewarding area of cancer treatment upon which we are about to embark. This is further exemplified below.

Current dramatic developments in the field of osteogenic sarcoma underscore the great benefits to be derived from in-depth clinical research with anticancer drugs. The cure rate for osteogenic sarcoma about 5 years ago ranged from 10% to 20%. Recently, applying the synthetic folic acid antagonist methotrexate at dose levels more than 100 times the safe maximum and then rescuing the patient with 5-formyl tetrahy-drofolate (citrovorum factor) has now increased the cure rate to over 60%.[102,103] Methotrexate is believed to inhibit dihydrofo-late reductase, which is needed for DNA and protein synthesis. The first clinical application of methotrexate was by Farber and colleagues[97] in 1948 against leukemia. The first investigation of methotrexate with citrovorum factor was described in 1953 by Goldin, who showed with experimental tumor systems that a methotrexate–citrovorum-factor rescue schedule could pro-duce a therapy superior to the single use of methotrexate.[97] Since the enzyme dihydrofolate reductase supplies 5-formyl tetrahydrofolate toxic effects of the high dosage with methotrexate can be reversed by the simple expedient of citrovorum-factor rescue. This technique has been unequivoc-ally demonstrated in osteogenic sarcoma by the Frei group.[103,171,325]

A major objective of the cancer conquest program in the United States is to develop new combinations of drugs that can be used to control and/or cure the slow-growing solid tumors that characterize cancer, for example, of the lung, the breast, the colon, and the ovary. The attack currently directed on these major clinical problems is based on the use of surgical and/or radiation treatment to remove most of the bulk cancer, with concurrent adjuvant chemotherapy for eradication of the mi-croscopic metastases. Already this approach is giving good results in breast cancer and gives hope of similar successes in lung[51] and colon cancer.[102] The extensive study led by Fischer and Carbone and colleagues[100] employing L-phenylalanine mustard (L-PAM) for adjuvant chemotherapy (with mastec-tomy) in patients with primary breast cancer (and positive axillary nodes) has established the effectiveness of this approach to treatment. Normally over 70% of such patients with axillary node metastases will expire from breast cancer. By the application of L-PAM, the recurrence rates at 18 months had been reduced from 33% to 3% for a tenfold decrease. Hopefully such treatment and the introduction of newer cancer chemotherapeutic agents in breast cancer will substantially increase the long-term survival rates. Various drug combinations are now under study for breast cancer, and the initial promising results—for example, with adriamycin and cyclophosphamide (cytoxan) by Jones[178] and with methotrexate-cyclophosphamide-5-fluorouracil (64% response rate)[291,33a,161a]—leave no doubt that this is the right route to the effective control of breast cancer and other solid tumor types. The rationale for treatment of cancer with drug combinations has been well documented by De Vita.[79,81] As he noted, a single-drug treatment would be an ideal method of cancer treatment, but several such drugs in combination are now known to give improved responses and survival rates. The whole concept of combination drug treatment for cancer seems most attractive and logical, as this would allow more chemical pathways to be interrupted simultaneously with less possibility of the emergence of a drug-resistant tumor line. Also, when a drug combination with nonoverlapping and different toxic effects is used, the result can be additive neoplastic cell kill without additive toxicity.[443] The four-drug treatments for acute lymphocytic leukemia and Hodgkin's disease are fine illustrations of this point.

Most of the currently available antineoplastic agents have in common a capacity to interfere with DNA synthesis. This means that the fraction of neoplastic cells initiating DNA synthesis at the time of drug treatment is especially important. In the early stages of neoplastic disease, the cells effect DNA syntheses at a rapid rate, leading to frequent cell division and a high growth rate. The high growth fraction of neoplastic cells decreases with time, and decreasing numbers of cells undergo DNA synthesis and division.[442] Rhoads[344] has calculated that to go from the original neoplastic disease to one weighing approximately 1 g, it would take about 1 year if the doubling time is a week. With a doubling time of 1 month, it would take 3–4 years, and if the tumor doubling time was quite slow, such as 3 months, it would take about 10 years. Generally this means that early neoplastic disease with a high growth fraction is more easily controlled by most currently available cancer chemotherapeutic drugs. As pointed out by Zubrod,[442] a most telling illustration of this effect is with Burkitt's lymphoma, in which nearly 100% of the neoplastic cells undergo division and a single dose of cytoxan (cyclophosphamide) cures 60% of the patients. For those neoplastic diseases with a smaller growth fraction, a combination of drugs acting through different mechanisms and at different points in the cell cycle is needed to effect complete cell kill. With old tumors such as colon and lung with growth fractions less than 5%, the rate of DNA synthesis is minimal, and these neoplasms are not very sensitive to currently available anticancer drugs. Thus diagnosis and the application of cancer chemotherapy at the earliest possible stage is imperative.

The discovery of new cancer chemotherapeutic agents with curative potential for the solid tumors with low growth fractions is a top-priority objective of the National Cancer Institute's Division of Cancer Treatment. Accordingly new screening systems have been introduced to assist in selecting such clinical candidates. The two principal evaluation systems now in use for this purpose are the B-16 melanoma (B1) and the Lewis lung carcinoma (LL). Both experimental tumor systems seem to have cell kinetics and other features related to the major types of human cancer. An extensive study of the correlations between experimental tumor systems used by the National Cancer Institute—particularly the LE, PS, and WA systems—and clinical effectiveness has been made by Venditti and Abbott.[409] Selection of the B1 and LL tumor systems was based on similar considerations.

Undoubtedly any number of substances can eventually be synthesized that will control and/or cure various types of solid tumors with low growth fractions. At present, we should be exceedingly enthusiastic about the prospects of uncovering many such useful cancer chemotherapeutic agents that already exist in plant and animal organisms. Such new biosynthetic products will also serve as useful starting points for further structural modification and the syntheses of potentially useful cancer chemotherapeutic drugs.

434

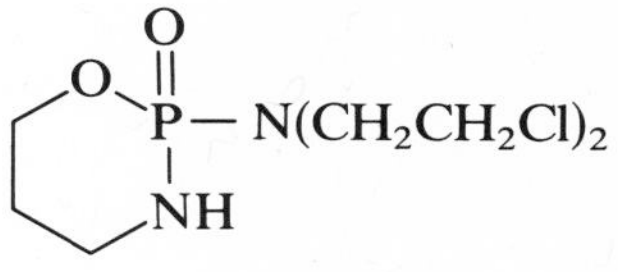

$$\text{O}$$
$$\|$$
$$\text{O}-\text{P}-\text{N(CH}_2\text{CH}_2\text{Cl)}_2$$
$$\overset{|}{\text{NH}}$$

7

Cyclophosphamide
(Cytoxan)

LE T/C >300, PS T/C 250
B1 T/C 162, LL T/C 180

434

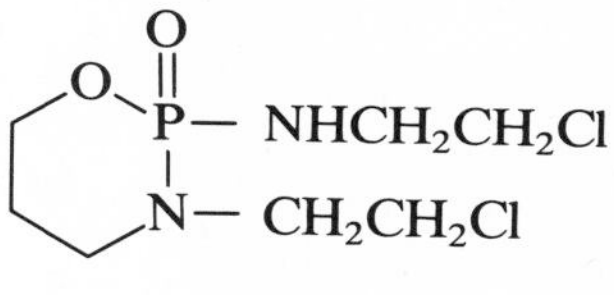

$$\text{O}$$
$$\|$$
$$\text{O}-\text{P}-\text{NHCH}_2\text{CH}_2\text{Cl}$$
$$\overset{|}{\text{N}}-\text{CH}_2\text{CH}_2\text{Cl}$$

8

Isophosphamide

LE T/C >300, PS T/C 300
B1 T/C 147, LL T/C 200

434

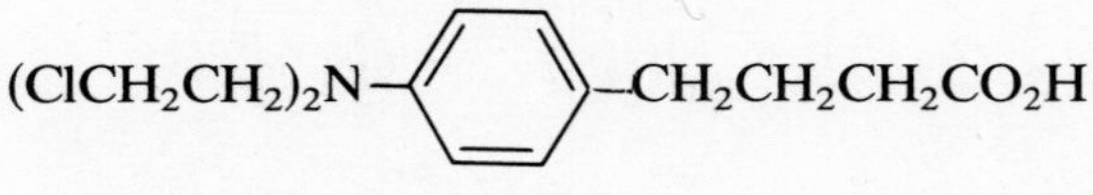

$$(ClCH_2CH_2)_2N-\overset{}{\underset{}{\bigcirc}}-CH_2CH_2CH_2CO_2H$$

9

Chloroambucil

LE T/C 131, PS T/C 198
B1 T/C 132, LL inactive

434

$$CH_3N(CH_2CH_2Cl)_2$$

10

N-Methyl nitrogen mustard
(Mechlorethamine, mustargen)

LE T/C 160, PS T/C 300
B1 T/C 185, LL inactive

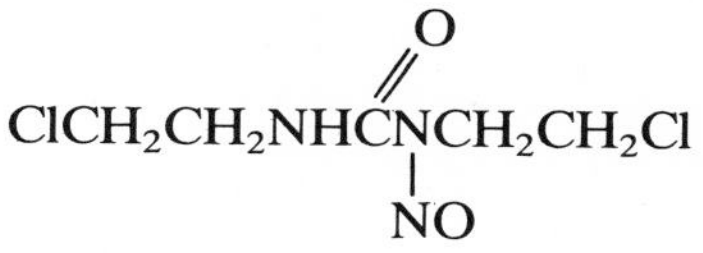

$$\text{ClCH}_2\text{CH}_2\text{NHCNCH}_2\text{CH}_2\text{Cl}$$

with carbonyl (O) above the C and NO below the N.

11

BCNU

LE T/C >300, PS T/C >300
B1 T/C 209, LL T/C 144

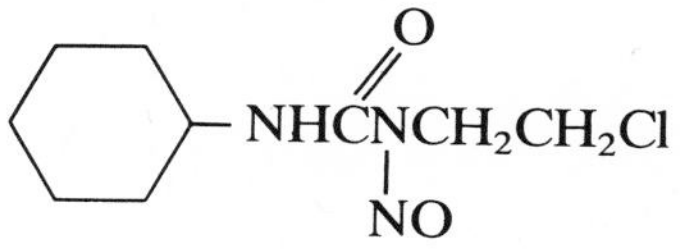

$$\text{NHCNCH}_2\text{CH}_2\text{Cl}$$

(cyclohexyl attached to NH, carbonyl O above C, NO below N)

12

CCNU

LE T/C >300, PS T/C 272
B1 T/C 300, LL T/C 130

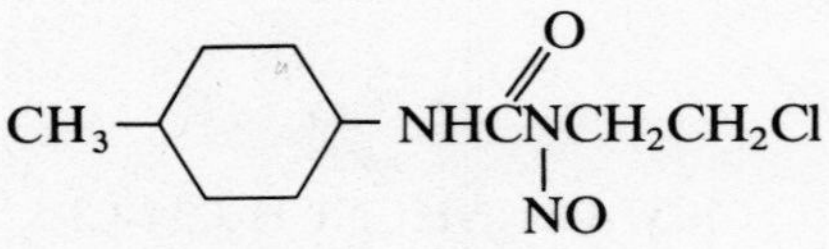

13

Methyl-CCNU

LE T/C >300, PS T/C 190
B1 T/C 234, LL >400

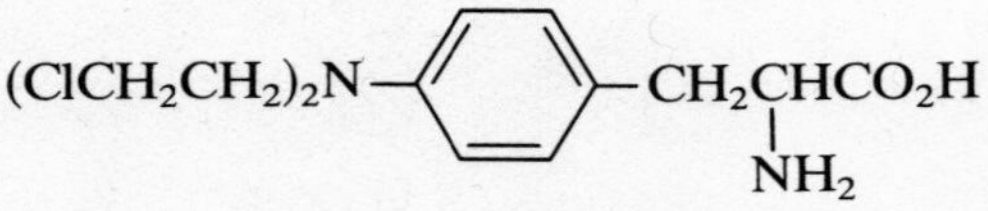

14

Mephalen

LE T/C 220, PS T/C 300
B1 T/C 205, LL inactive

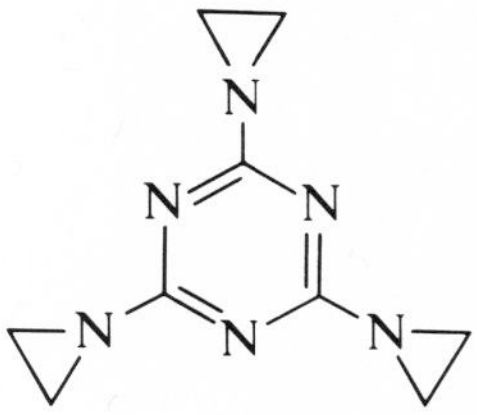

15

Triethylene melamine

LE T/C 168, PS T/C 271
B1 T/C 130, LL inactive

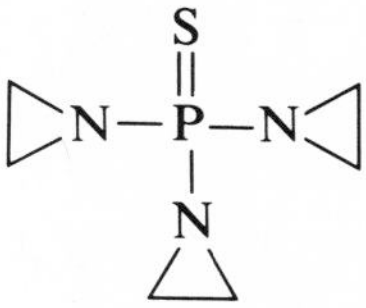

16

Thiotepa

LE T/C 180, PS T/C 131
B1 inactive, LL T/C 130

17

Cytosine arabinoside
(Ara-C, cytarabine)

LE T/C 200, PS T/C 221
B1 T/C 160, LL T/C 137

18

5-Fluorouracil
(5-FU, FU)

LE T/C 180, PS T/C 220
B1 T/C 140, LL inactive

19

5-FUDR

LE T/C 152, PS T/C 255
B1 T/C 138, LL T/C 128

20

Ftorafur

LE T/C 154, PS, B1 and
LL inactive

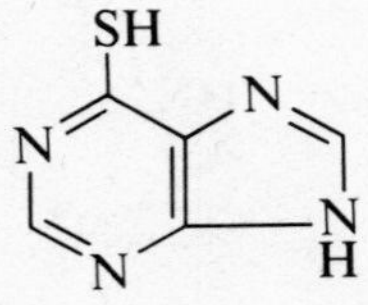

21

6-Mercaptopurine
(6-MP)

LE T/C 160, PS, B1 and
LL inactive

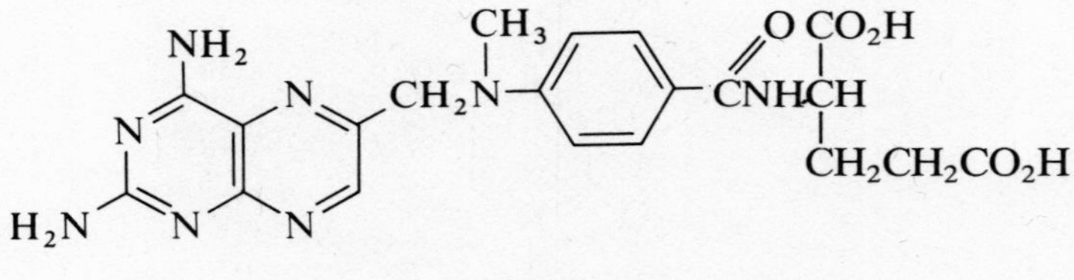

22

Methotrexate
(MTX)

LE T/C 205, PS T/C >300
B1 and LL inactive

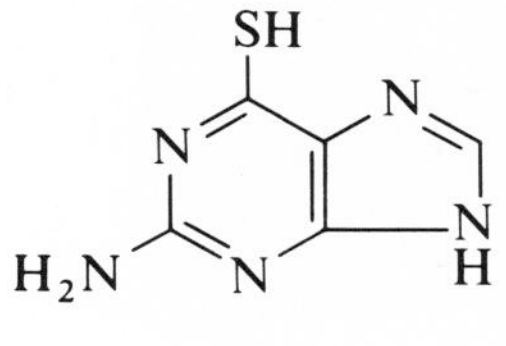

23

Thioquanine
(6-TG)

LE T/C 163, PS T/C 132
B1 and LL inactive

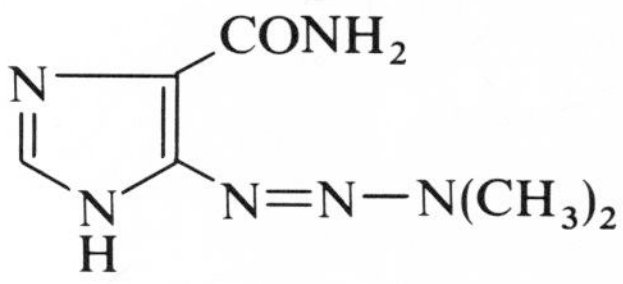

24

5-(3,3-Dimethyl-1-triazenol)-
imidazole-4-carboxamide
(DTC, dacarbazine)

LE T/C 160, PS T/C 154
B1 T/C 145, LL inactive

$$\overset{\displaystyle O}{\overset{\displaystyle \|}{NH_2CNHOH}}$$

25

Hydroxyurea

LE T/C 278, PS T/C 150
B1 inactive, LL T/C 129

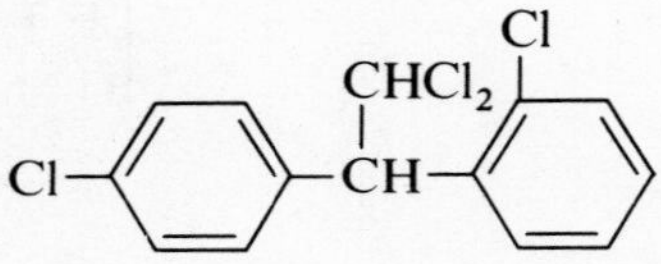

25a

Mitotane

$$\overset{\displaystyle O}{\overset{\displaystyle \|}{CH_3OSOCH_2(CH_2)_2CH_2O}}\overset{\displaystyle O}{\overset{\displaystyle \|}{SOCH}}$$

26

Busulfan
(Myleran)

LE, PS, B1 and LL inactive

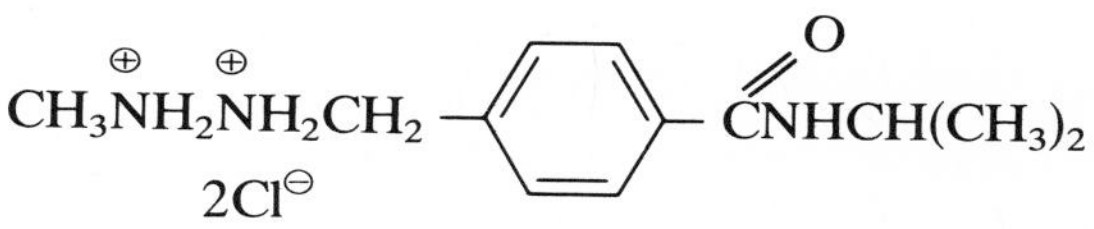

$$\overset{\oplus}{CH_3NH_2}\overset{\oplus}{NH_2}CH_2 -\!\!\!\!\bigcirc\!\!\!\!- \overset{O}{\overset{\|}{C}}NHCH(CH_3)_2$$

$$2Cl^{\ominus}$$

27

Procarbazine hydrochloride

LE T/C 152, PS T/C 160
B1 T/C 132, LL inactive

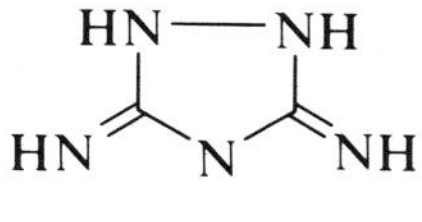

$$HN\!-\!NH$$
$$HN\diagdown{\underset{N}{}}\diagup NH$$

28

Guanazole

LE T/C 167, PS T/C 145
B1 and LL inactive

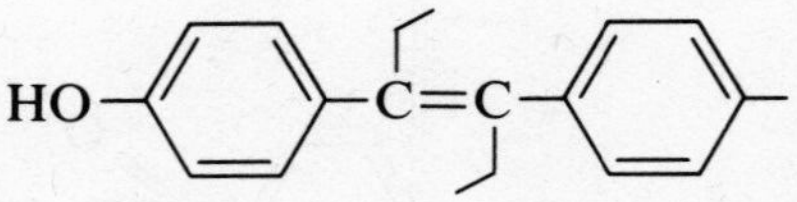

29

Diethylstilbestrol
(DES)

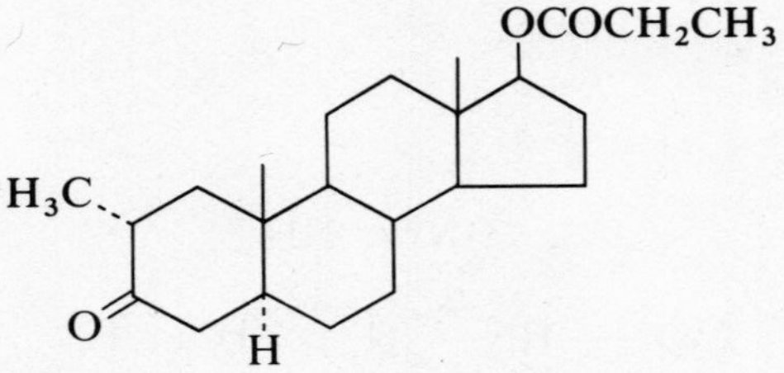

30

Dromostanolone propionate
(Drolban)

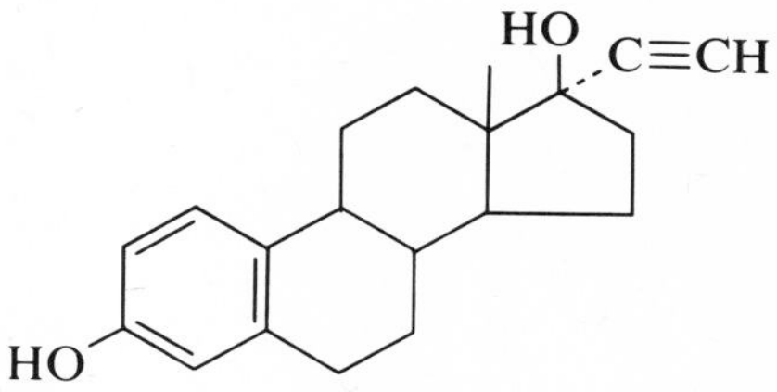

31

Ethinyl estradiol

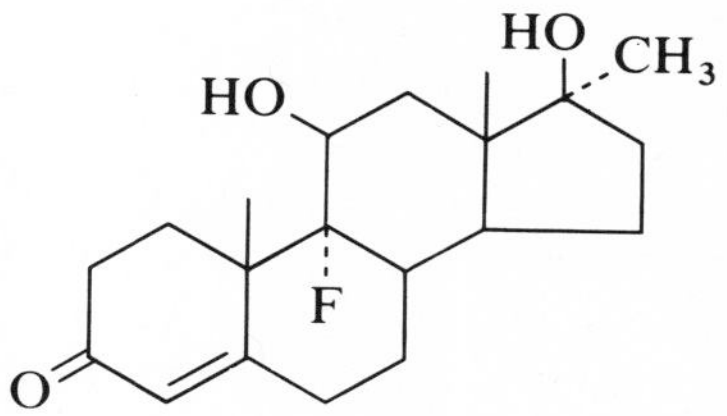

32

Fluoxymesterone

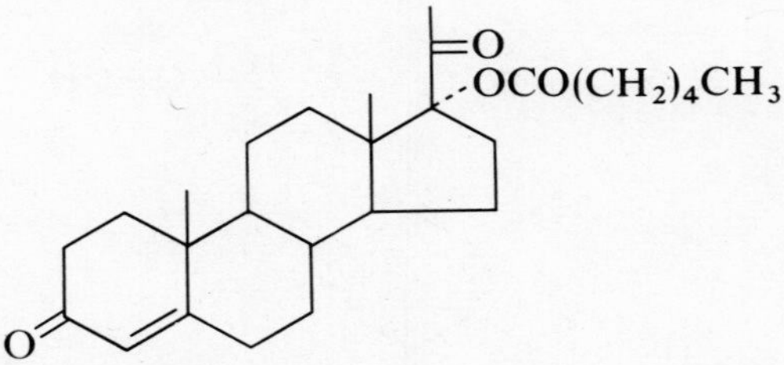

33

Hydroxyprogesterone caproate

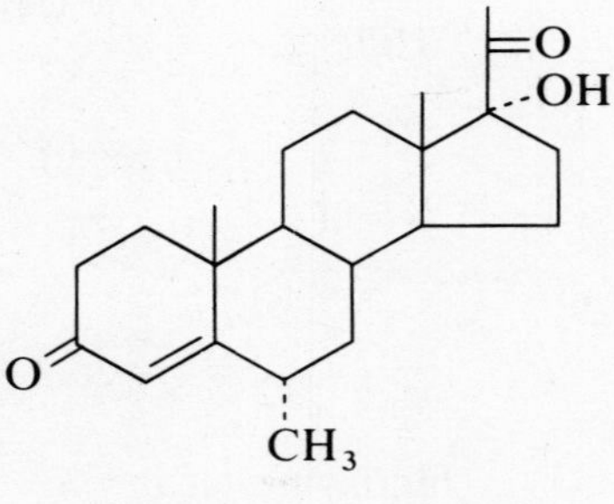

34

Medroxyprogesterone

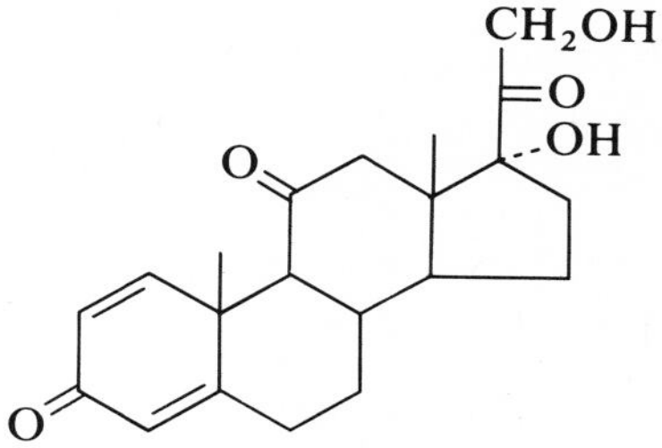

35

Prednisone

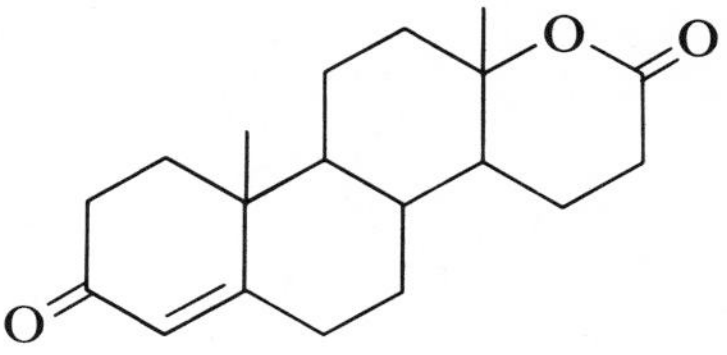

36

Testolactone
(Teslac)

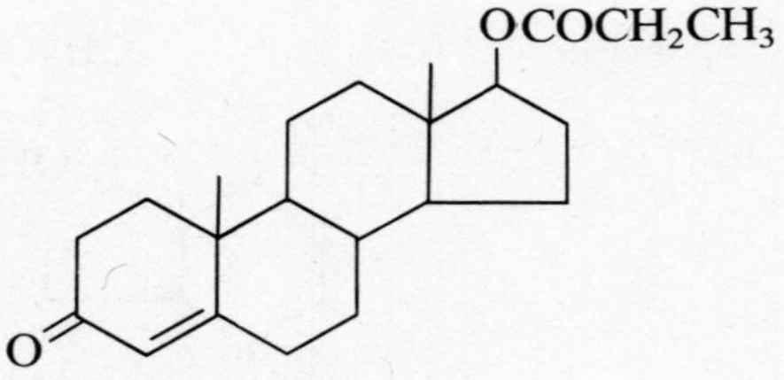

37

Testosterone propionate

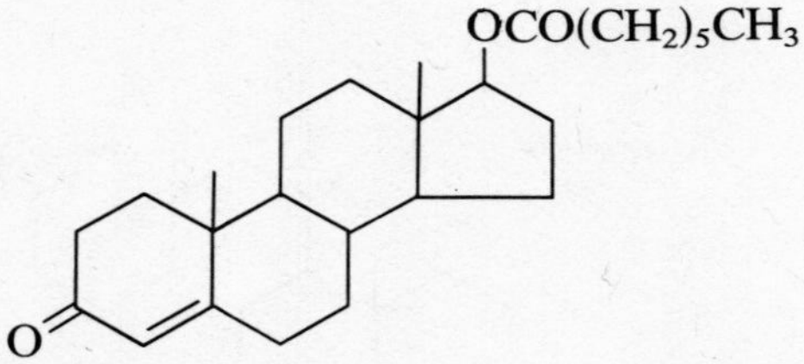

38

Testosterone enanthate

Naturally Occurring Antineoplastic and Cytotoxic Agents

> *"Instead of assuming that the mediaeval pharmacist was a benighted fool, we might wonder whether there was not sometimes a justification for his strange procedure."*
>
> *G. Sarton*[144]

The earliest applications in cancer treatment of materials derived from natural products probably began with the development of man's reasoning abilities. The general use of medicinal plants has been known for at least 60,000 years. Remains of a human body and plants placed in an Iraqi cave at that time have recently been found. Seven of the eight pollens discovered were identified as from medicinal plants.[342] The Egyptian medical papyri, particularly the Ebers Papyrus of approximately 1550 B.C.,[91] describe the use of plant materials for afflictions assumed to be cancer. Such recorded references begin with the Chinese Shen-Nung of the period 2838–2698 B.C., but these materials were probably well known much earlier. Indeed some of this information still forms an integral part of traditional Chinese medical treatment, and a variety of plant extracts are currently in use as supportive measures for contemporary cancer treatment.[299] In this regard, modern development in China of medicinal agents from plants is greatly influenced by Mao's view that "Chinese medicine and pharmacology are a great treasure house and must be explored and raised to a higher level." While a member of the U.S. Academy of Sciences medical and pharmacology delegation to the People's Republic of China in 1974, this writer was pleased to see that quotation prominently displayed in the Peking Institute of Materia Medica, where new cancer chemotherapeutic agents are being developed.

From the valuable and comprehensive survey of plants employed in primitive cancer treatment begun by Hartwell[142,143] in the 1950's and completed in 1971,[139a] we know that 17 medical works containing plant extract treatments for cancer were written prior to the year 50 B.C. In the same time frame Hippocrates (460–349 B.C.) may have been the first to use the word *carcinoma*. And the use of an arsenic paste for the treatment of cancer had already been described in the Ebers Papyrus.[91] From the second century A.D., 18 works have been preserved describing the use of plants in cancer treatment. Another 45 summaries of plants for cancer treatment are known for the period to about A.D. 1000, 50 to about A.D. 1300 and 95 more proceeding on into the 19th century. Fortunately, because of the remarkable preservation and location[143] of these valuable accounts of primitive medicine and more recent collections,[143,144] we can estimate that more than 3,000 different plant species have found use in the primitive treatment of cancer. Many additional plant species are mentioned in letters written to the National Cancer Institute. These include some 600 letters received at the time of former Secretary of State John Foster Dulles's fatal struggle with cancer.[144]

Other early approaches to cancer treatment include the caustic pastes and cautery of Hippocrates and the first cancer surgery (including mastectomies), performed by Celsus in the first century A.D.[124] One of the first recorded attempts to use a single substance for cancer chemotherapy is attributed to Lissauer.[245] In 1865, he reported remissions in chronic leukemias resulting from the use of potassium arsenite (Fowler's solution). Unfortunately this first step in modern cancer chemotherapy does not seem to have received much attention, but such advances probably did move Gurin (in Kiev) in 1908 to write, "let the chemical treatment of tumors meet not the poison of venomous doubt and cynicism, but the blissful joy of hope."[235] Similarly, implications of the bone marrow and lymphoid effects of mustard gas on soldiers slain in World War I were not connected with possibilities for leukemia treatment until World War II.[351] The result was a clinical trial of nitrogen mustard against leukemia in 1942. These war-effort–related investigations of bis(2-chloroethyl)amine were eventually published by several groups in 1946. A well-documented and interesting account, especially of highlights in synthetic anticancer drug development, has been prepared by Burchenal.[43] In the 1940's, the real impetus that led to present-day advances in both synthetic and biosynthetic cancer chemotherapeutic agents was taking place almost simultaneously. Advances in the synthetic and biosynthetic approaches have been mutually stimulating and each has inspired renewed efforts.

In 1944, Kendall[153] reported the application of his newly discovered cortisone against murine lymphosarcoma. Further development of this important lead led to the synthetic modification prednisone now used in many types of combination cancer chemotherapy. One of the first examples of drug combinations for cancer treatment was probably that of cortisone with methotrexate described by Bernard and colleagues in 1951.[27]

In the field of plant biosynthetic products, the clinical activity of colchicine was already known in the 1940's. Subsequently deacetyl-*N*-methyl-colchicine (cholcemide) has been used to treat both human leukemias and human lymphomas.[242] A number of plants contain colchicine; one of the most common sources is the meadow saffron, *Colchicum autumnale* L. (Liliaceae). Interestingly toxic properties of the *Colchicum* genus was described by Dioscorides in A.D. 78.[62] The first isolation of colchicine was described by Pelleter and Caventou[293] in 1820, and a pure specimen was obtained by Zeisel in 1883.[440] *Podophyllum peltatum* L. (Berberidaceae) is another plant with a long history of use in primitive medicine and was already under investigation in the 1940's by Hartwell at the National Cancer Institute.[143] These pioneering studies led to recognition of the cytotoxic properties of podophyllotoxin and more recently to preparation of 4′-demethyl-epipodophyllotoxin-β-D-thienylidene-glucoside (**94**) of current interest, for example, in treatment of intracranial neoplasms.[93,281,374] By 1958, the characterization and application of the *Vinca rosea* alkaloids vinblastine (**105**)[72,73,74,282] and vincristine (**104**)[277,386] were already well under way.[173,277]

The development of clinically useful anticancer agents from microorganisms began with Fleming's[101] discovery of penicillin in 1929. However, the implications of this discovery for the chemotherapy of infectious diseases did not gain impetus until further development by Chain and Florey in 1940.[55] The same year Waksman and Woodruff[414] reported the actinomycins' antibiotic activity and their pronounced toxicity. But it was not until 1952 that Schulte[365] employed actinomycin B against Hodgkin's disease. Farber[95,96,97] reported additional work in 1955. These very encouraging results with the actinomycins set the stage for the uncovering of the series of antibiotic antineoplastic agents made available during the 1960's. Those with proven clinical cancer chemotherapeutic properties include the mitomycins (1959),[381] daunomycin (1964),[82,355] mithramycin (1965),[16,337] the bleomycins (1966),[275,391,406,407] adriamycin (1969),[10,83,113,355] and carminomycin I (1974).[35,108]

The isolation of cancer chemotherapeutic agents from animal sources began to be successful in terms of clinical agents in the 1950's. Discovery of the previously unknown marine animal β-D-arabinosyl nucleosides spongouridine (**39**) and spongothymidine (**40**) by Bergmann and Feeney[25,26] led to the synthesis of cytosine arabinoside[152] (ara-C, **17**) in 1959.[421] In the same time period, guinea pig serum was found to inhibit murine lymphosarcoma, and this discovery was followed by the isolation and clinical application (acute leukemia) of the enzyme L-asparaginase.[41,49,191]

The systematic development of drugs for cancer chemotherapy (and for other medical problems) from plant and animal products has been seriously slowed by a general lack of understanding of the great potential. This situation has been

39

Spongouridine

40

Spongothymidine

aggravated by the paucity of organic chemists being trained for such very challenging endeavors and the lack of necessary financial support for personnel (and laboratories). Undoubtedly the many unethical and outright fraudulent[18] business practices connected with the merchandising of plant remedies in the early part of this century diverted attention from the real promise. Fortunately Shear, under the Office of Cancer Investigation, U.S. Public Health Service (at Harvard University), had the foresight in the mid-1930's to begin a screening program utilizing bacterial polysaccharides against murine sarcoma 37.[50,117] This early screening program was terminated in 1953 and by that time had included over 3,000 compounds and several hundred plants.[50] However, it was rekindled in earnest by the National Cancer Institute (NCI) in the 1953–55 period.[94,351]

The NCI's chemotherapy program formally began in July 1953, when Congress directed the institute to explore the practicality of a broad program focused on the chemotherapy of acute leukemia. In April 1955, the Cancer Chemotherapy National Service Center (CCNSC) was established, and the NCI increased its grant support for all areas of chemotherapy to approximately $3 million. For the July 1955 fiscal year, the congressional appropriation for chemotherapy was increased to $5 million, and the first contracts were let for four major screening centers. The first major chemical effort of the National Cancer Institute was in the steroid hormone area, and in 1956 $5 million of the total $19 million appropriated for chemotherapy was set aside for this endeavor. Elsewhere in the 1950's, screening programs for cancer chemotherapeutic agents were under way, for example, at the Chester Beatty Research Institute in London, the Children's Cancer Research Foundation in Boston, the Institute of Clinical and Experimental Oncology in Moscow, the Sloan-Kettering Institute in New York City, and the University of Tokyo.

The survey of microorganisms for anticancer agents begun by Umezawa at the University of Tokyo in 1951[405] had already yielded sarkomycin by 1953, and the Sloan-Kettering program with antibiotics began to look hopeful. At the NCI, the large-scale screening of synthetic compounds against experimental neoplastic diseases was begun in December 1955, and this program was quickly enlarged to encompass microorganism culture filtrates ("beers"). The latter approach was quickly expanded, and by 1957 it was known that about 1% of microorganism beers would significantly inhibit experimental tumor systems in mice.[94]

A recommendation that the CCNSC of the NCI should begin a broad screening program involving plants was made by Hartwell very early in the program. In a memorandum dated December 17, 1957, he suggested beginning with the Compositae, the Euphorbiaceae, the Labiatae, the Leguminosae, the Liliaceae, and the Umbelliferae.[139] This writer had been stimulated by Hartwell's early studies of podophyllotoxin[301,302] and by 1957 was anxious to begin an investigation of plant anticancer constituents at the University of Maine. In October and November of that year, this interest was expressed to Ross in the CCNSC.[297] Because of Hartwell's survey, it was decided in December 1957 to begin a collaborative anticancer constituents survey of the Labiatae family.[350] Arrangements for the first Labiatae plant collections were made by Jones of the U.S. Department of Agriculture (USDA), and the first shipments of plant specimens were received at Maine in the spring of 1958. In September 1958, our first shipment of extracts from Labiatae species was sent to the CCNSC screening laboratories. However, because of the virtual lack of financial support, this part of the program remained barely viable until about 1966. Late in 1957, Herz at Florida State University agreed to continue his earlier studies of the Compositae on a collaborative basis with the CCNSC. Similarly Kupchan, then at the University of Wisconsin, and Cava, then at Ohio State University, expressed an interest in beginning chemical studies of other plant families.[350]

In the summer of 1957, Hartwell transferred to the CCNSC staff to supervise the natural products programs. The search for plant antineoplastic agents then began in earnest, and some 600 extracts from plants collected in the western hemisphere and Africa by the Eastern Utilization Research and Development Division of the USDA (during their search for sapogenin steroid precursors) were screened along with several hundred more sent by Caldwell at the University of Arizona.[351] Several promising results came from this initial screening of plant extracts, and one important outgrowth was the later isolation and characterization of camptothecin by the Wall group from one of the original USDA extracts.[417]

By 1959 the plant program looked very hopeful and by 1964 was well underway. At that time substantial NCI contract support was provided to Kupchan's group to isolate antineoplastic and cytotoxic constituents from plant extracts with a confirmed level of activity discovered in the National Cancer Institute plant collection, extraction, and screening programs. The plant collections were made under contract (beginning in 1960) between the National Cancer Institute and the U.S. Department of Agriculture (first under Erlanson and then Q. Jones). In 1960 formal arrangements were also made with Caldwell (University of Arizona) and Wall (USDA) for providing plant extracts. Next arrangements were made with laboratories in India (1962) and Australia (1963). Extraction and screening was performed under contract with the Wisconsin Alumni Research Foundation. In recent years the USDA collections (and field botany) has been directed by Perdue and were maintained at about 1,000 new species per year for a number of years. In 1973–1974 the rate was increased to about 8,000 but is currently being substantially reduced.

In the mid-1960's isolation contracts were awarded to Wall (Research Triangle Institute) and Caldwell. In recent years the latter program has been managed by Cole. The contract program, begun with Kupchan at the University of Wisconsin, was transferred with his move to the University of Virginia.[199,200] Several years ago, National Cancer Institute laboratories for the plant program were established with Farnsworth at the University of Illinois. A very enlightening summary of the screening procedures and advances in this program to about 1968 has been prepared by Hartwell and Abbott.[145] Additionally, a considerable number of governmental, university, and private laboratories all over the world are now collaborating with the National Cancer Institute's natural products program on an informal or NIH grant basis.

Independent plant-extract screening programs have also been under way, for example, in the Soviet Union at the Moscow Institute of Clinical and Experimental Oncology and in the People's Republic of China at the Institutes of Materia Medica in Peking and Shanghai.[299] The NCI fermentation program has been conducted primarily in the NCI contract laboratories at the Bristol, Parke Davis, Pfizer, and Upjohn companies and at the Michigan Department of Health. The program is now carried out principally at the Parke Davis and Upjohn companies. In addition to the institute directed by Umezawa at the University of Tokyo, the Institute of New Antibiotics in Moscow, directed by Gauze, has been especially productive in discovery of new anticancer agents in microorganisms. The success of both groups is based on great expertise in microbiology and organic chemistry.

In 1965, Zubrod was given the most challenging assignment of reorganizing the CCNSC into a comprehensive cancer chemotherapy program, and following passage of the National Cancer Act of 1971, the program was expanded to cover other modalities of cancer therapy and restructured into the present division of cancer treatment. With brilliant leadership, Zubrod continued to strengthen the NCI cancer chemotherapy and treatment programs until he left in May 1974 to direct the University of Miami Cancer Center. In the summer of 1974, De Vita was selected to continue direction of the NCI Cancer Treatment Division.

In the 1965–66 period, our group began a new colloborative program with the Drug Research and Development Branch of the NCI involving the first systematic investigation of arthropods[309] and marine organisms[304] for anticancer and cytotoxic components. The processing of animal extracts has steadily increased from about 400 in 1967 to 2,000 in 1974. Generally we have found almost 10% of marine animal extracts to show a confirmed level of activity against the NCI's P-388 lymphocytic leukemia and/or KB cell line. Otherwise the major natural-products areas—namely, the lower and higher plants— have continued to receive major emphasis.

About 1968, the overall total of plant extracts screened amounted to 40,000, but because of duplication and multiple extracts from the same plant, this number represented a much smaller number of actual plant species. However, it was clear by 1968 that some 3.5% of plant species would give extracts with a confirmed level of antineoplastic or cytotoxic activity.[145] Initially the screening of fermentation beers was at a high level and in 1958 amounted to some 30,000 such filtrates compared to 10,000 synthetic compounds.[351] Meanwhile the NCI's screening of fermentation products has continued to decrease. By 1966, the number of such extracts amounted to approximately 4,000 per year and has steadily decreased to a low of some 700 in 1974. The NCI's screening of plant extracts averaged about 4,000 per year from 1966 to 1971 and for the next 2 years was increased to about 10,000 per year, with a drop to slightly under 6,000 in 1974. The screening[116] of synthetic compounds by the NCI remained at about 8,000–10,000 per year over the period 1958–71, whereupon it was increased over the next 3 years to a high of nearly 40,000 in 1974.

The latter increase was made possible by passage of the National Cancer Act in 1971, which increased the United States cancer budget in 1971 to $228 million. From 1972 to 1975 the budget was increased respectively to $378 million, $432 million, $589 million, and $699 million. However, of the 1975 budget only about $60 million was spent on the NCI's intramural research programs.[363] Most serious has been the continued inability to provide more than a few million dollars each year for discovery of new cancer chemotherapeutic drugs by the NCI Division of Cancer Treatment. At the same time, continued (1971–76) delays in the approval of the NCI budgets because of disagreements in the federal executive and legislative branches over the total Health, Education, and Welfare budget, combined with a series of NCI budget impoundments by the Office of Management and Budget have seriously impeded progress. Some conception of these budgetary problems can be gained by the realization that each time a new fiscal year begins and the NCI budget has not been approved, the institute must operate at the prior year's level. Thus in 1974, with inflation at a 12% annual rate, this meant a comparable decrease in the program for that period. While the United States annual rate of inflation fell back to 7% in 1975, severe understaffing and budgetary limitations in the NCI Division of Cancer Treatment meant a drastic curtailment of exploratory screening programs for cancer chemotherapeutic drugs in 1975–76. Needless to say, this is a tragic event for the future. The NCI Drug Research and Development program—most expertly led, under extremely challenging circumstances (incredible understaffing), by Wood and Engle—has been exceptionally productive. A substantial number of the new biosynthetic natural products described in the sequel, as well as most of the clinically effective synthetic compounds, have been developed by this most important program.

Some realization of the amount of exploratory screening that is necessary to the discovery of a potentially useful anti-cancer drug can be obtained if one considers that some 3,000–4,000 synthetic compounds must be evaluated before one candidate for clinical trial is obtained. Generally about 1 clinical candidate in 10 proves really effective, so it is necessary to screen about 30,000 compounds to obtain one clinically useful drug.[360] There is nothing unusual about this yield, as similar numbers are required with certain other types of medical problems and even for the discovery of a good pesticide. Obviously it would be in the best public interest to speed up the input in the screening of both synthetic and biosynthetic compounds.

The vast supply of potential cancer chemotherapeutic drugs available from plants and animals has for practical purposes been essentially untapped. About 300,000 plants are known, but enough funds have been available in the NCI program to evaluate (since 1958) only about 10% of this number. With regard to soil microorganisms, less than 40,000 fermentation beers from actinomycetaceae, streptomycetaceas, and some bacteria have been screened. Obviously there must be millions of such microorganism species, so the potential here is enormous. Similarly, just among the the marine invertebrates, there are about 1 million known species, and if one considers the fishes, there are over 25,000 known species. In the arthropod area, the insect class Insecta alone comprises about 1 million different species. We also now have definite evidence that in addition to the plants and soil microorganisms, the marine animals and arthropods show great promise of providing us with new and structurally novel clinical agents for cancer chemotherapy.

No organic chemist or other scientist is now able to design the single substance that would be most effective for the chemotherapeutic control of human cancer. Therefore for some time to come, such exploratory screening of biosynthetic and synthetic compounds must be continued. At the same time, it will be necessary to proceed as rapidly as resources permit with the synthesis of compounds reflecting logical extensions of existing structural leads and with the isolation and structural determination of new naturally occurring antineoplastic agents.

The new biosynthetic products will continue to provide some of the best means by which great advances will be made possible in cancer treatment. Such substances synthesized by plant and animal organisms are of such complexity and bear such unique design that no one can predict in advance the details of the great wealth of drugs for the control of cancer still waiting to be discovered in natural products. At the same time, each new biosynthetic product with anticancer activity serves as a useful starting point for structural modification and other synthetic efforts. Unless a complex natural product has been shown to have useful antineoplastic activity or other medically useful properties, an organic chemist would not usually undertake the years of effort and challenge necessary to synthesize such a compound. This point has been succinctly made by Venditti and Abbott[409] in their commentary "unhampered by technical difficulties, nature continues to produce novel structures."

Many of the great successes in medicine in terms of chemotherapeutic treatment have involved either using a natural product, such as quinine, penicillin, tetracycline, or reserpine, or substances obtained by suitable modifications of other biosynthetic products. There is every reason to believe that a variety of exceptionally useful cancer chemotherapeutic drugs will continue to arise based on biosynthetic products and synthetic compounds systematically uncovered in the NCI and other such exploratory screening programs. Indeed this observer is quite certain that cancer will be controlled and cured by this means long before the fundamental cell chemistry and biology of cancer are understood.

Chapter 3

Higher Plant Terpenoids

Plants are phenomenally adept at biosyntheses of complex and potentially useful terpenoids. A considerable number of species from plant families rich in terpenoids, such as the Compositae, have been used in primitive cancer treatment from a pre-Christian period of unknown length. The possibilities for isolation of anticancer agents from the Compositae—and, for example, the Euphorbiaceae[159]—were anticipated at least 20 years ago by Hartwell at the U.S. National Cancer Institute (NCI), as noted in Chapter 2. Subsequent investigations of Compositae, particularly by Hertz and Kupchan, have led to a number of new sesquiterpenes capable of substantially inhibiting ($ED_{50} < 10 \mu g/ml$) the KB cell line. The application of this *in vitro* screening technique for bioassay markedly enhanced the facility with which such cytotoxic substances can be isolated. Unfortunately, in a significant number of cases, the cytotoxicity has not been translated into *in vivo* activity against the NCI's lymphocytic leukemia P388 (the PS system, significant activity ≥ 125 T/C), Walker carcinosarcoma 256 (the WA system, significant activity ≤ 42 T/C), or lymphoid leukemia L1210 (the LE system, significant activity ≥ 125 T/C). Because the main emphasis of this volume is on the potential of biosynthetic products for cancer chemotherapy, the discussion here will be limited to those terpenoids with *in vivo* antineoplastic activity. However, all of those available in the literature with cytotoxic activity have been listed in the tabular survey of Volume 2. The same format has been followed in each subsequent chapter.

The C_{15} sesquiterpenoid alcohol farnesol is believed to be a biological precursor of the sesquiterpenes. Almost every reasonable cyclization and rearrangement conceivable for farnesol is reflected in the sesquiterpenes, and a number of these possibilities, as highly oxygenated derivatives, have been found to be cytotoxic and/or antineoplastic agents. The eudesmane skeleton appears in the unusual *seco*-eudesmanolides eriolangin (**41**) and eriolanin (**42**) from *Eriophyllum lanatum* Forbes (Compositae).[203] Vernolepin (**43**) is an unusual emanolide from *Vernolia hymenolepis* A. Rich. (Compositae).[214,219] The somewhat related iridoid lactone, allamandin (**44**) from the Apocynaceae species *Allamanda cathartica* Linn., provides an example from a plant family better known for its alkaloid constituents.[212]

The sesquiterpene hydrocarbon germacrane appears in the germacranolide lactones represented by structures **45** through **52**. Each was isolated by the Kupchan group[211] from a Compositae, and liatrin (**49**) was found to possess an interesting level of PS activity. Three other cytotoxic germacranolides have been found by Doskotch and co-workers in the Magnoliaceae plant *Liriodendron tulipifera* L.[85,86]

Three sesquiterpene lactones with the guaiane carbon framework have been located that possess solid tumor activity. The tumor inhibitory activity reported by the Cole group[401] for ambrosin (**53**, Asteraceae) is surprisingly high. Of eight cytotoxic lactones isolated from *Eupatorium rotundifolium* L. (Compositae), the two given by structures **54** and **55** were found active in the WA system. The pseudoguaiane carbon network corresponds to a one carbon shift of the cyclopentane methyl group into the guaiane ring juncture. A number of such pseudoguaianolides are known.[156,346]

Our group has found the common sneeze-weed[170] of Oregon, *Helenium autumnale* L. Var. *Montanum* (Nutt.) Fern. (Compositae), to give extracts with a good level of PS activity,

203

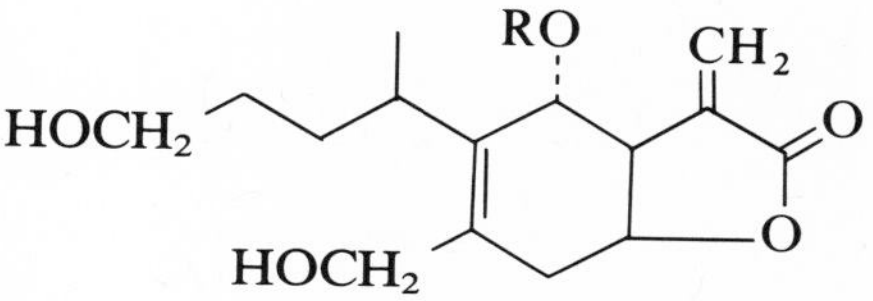

41, R = COC=C

CH$_3$ H

CH$_3$

Eriolangin

42, R = COC=CH$_2$

CH$_3$

Eriolanin

PS active

214
219

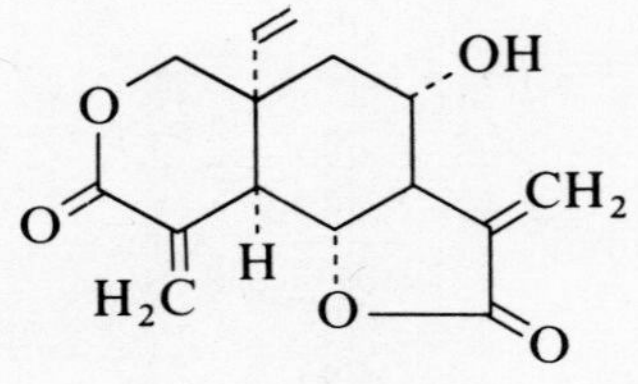

43

Vernolepin

WA T/C 46 (10 mg/kg)

212

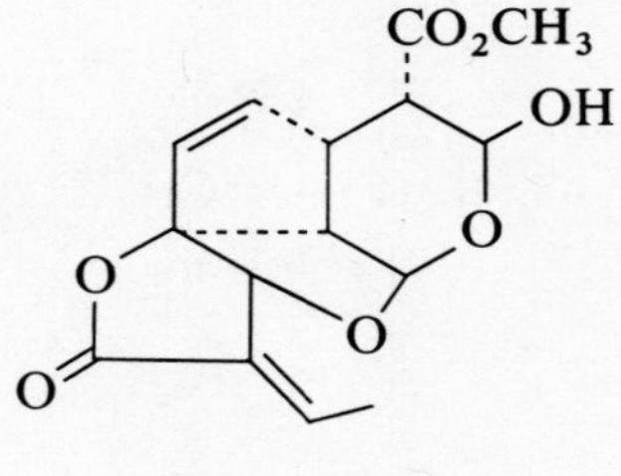

44

Allamandin

PS active

239

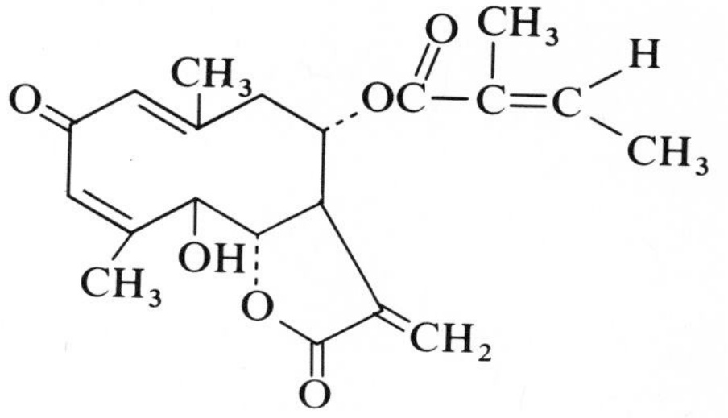

45

Molephantinin

WA active

227

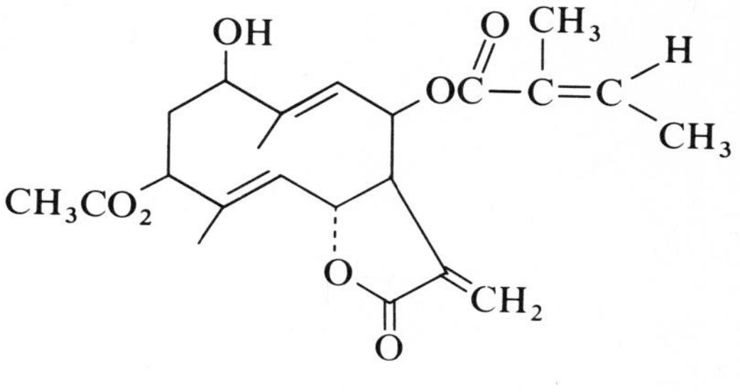

46

Eupacunin

PS active

216

47, R = COC=C
Eupaserrin

48, R = COC=C
Deacetyleupaserrin

PS active

211

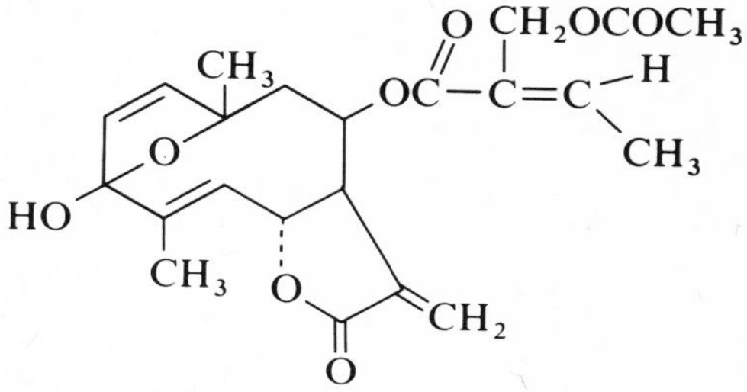

49

Liatrin

PS T/C 157 (5–8 mg/kg)

203

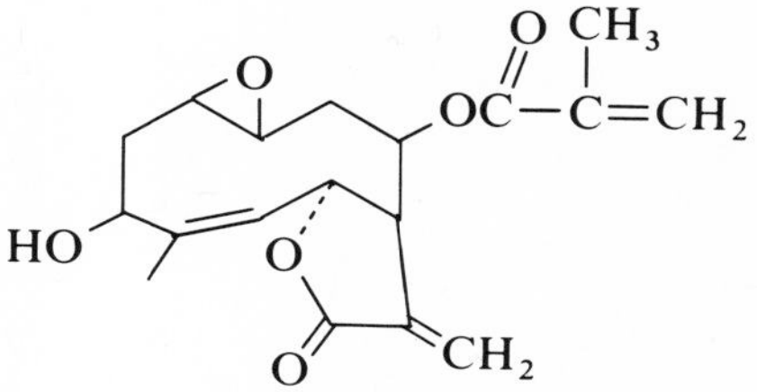

50

Erioflorin

PS active

202
214

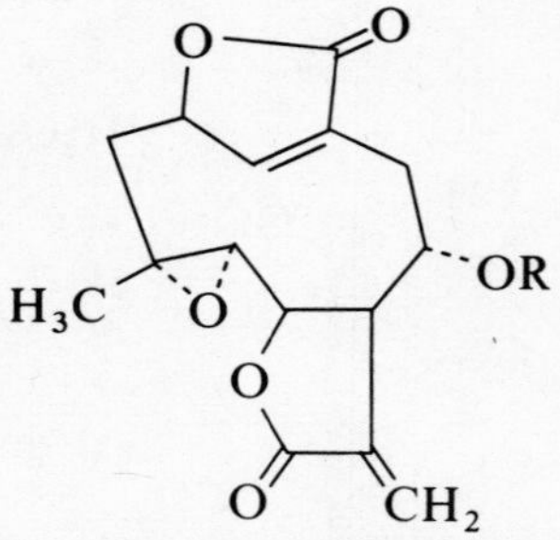

51, R = $-COCH{=}C(CH_3)_2$

Elephantin

WA T/C 12 (100 mg/kg)

52, R = $-CO\overset{CH_3}{\overset{|}{C}}{=}CH_2$

Elephantopin

PS T/C 140 (40 mg/kg)

401

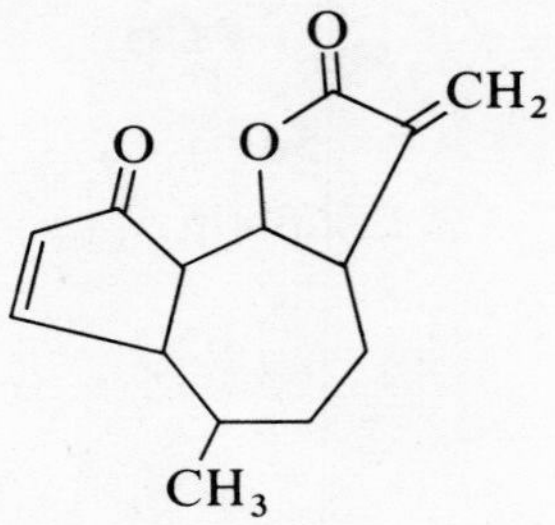

53

Ambrosin

PS T/C 180 (35 mg/kg)

222

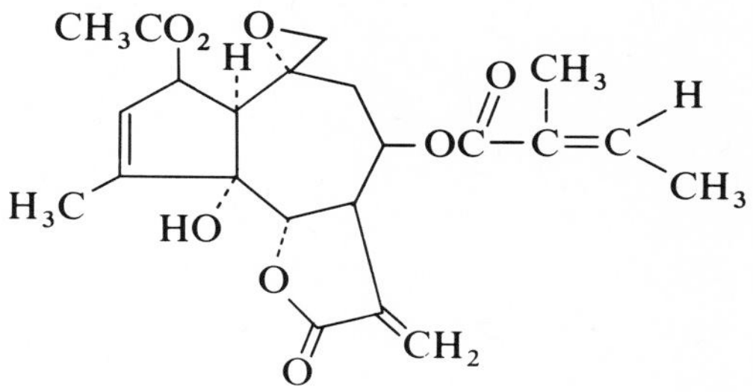

54

Euparotin acetate

WA T/C 12 (100 mg/kg)

222

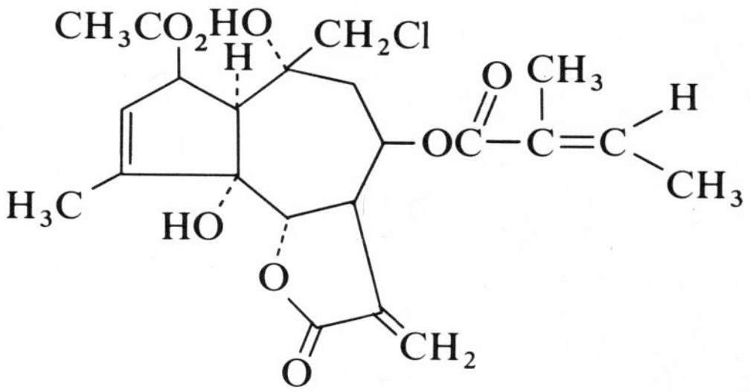

55

Eupachlorin acetate

WA active

and the active agent was found to be the pseudoguaianolide helenalin (**56**).[303,411] The NCI's P388 cell line was applied to isolating active components of *Bailyea multiradiata* (Compositae), and we found several of the constituents—particularly radiatin (**57**), fastigilin C (**58**), and multigilin (**59**)—to possess promising PS activity.[312] Similarly the Herz group[157] has reported significant LE activity for hymenoflorin (**60**) and PS activity for paucin (**61**). Both lactones **60** and **61** were isolated from a Rocky Mountain alpine Compositae. Most of the Compositae investigated so far are from lower elevations and in most cases semitropical regions.

Some of the structural features necessary for *in vivo* activity among the sesquiterpene lactones are readily apparent. The extended π-electron systems involving lactones and carbonyl groups are quite obvious.[309,214] However, in most cases it may also be necessary to have an angelic acid ester side-chain or similar α,β-unsaturated carbonyl system. This view is shared by Kupchan. Another interesting possibility for *in vivo* activity might be glucoside formation as evidenced by paucin (**61**). Indeed some of the more readily available cytotoxic sesquiterpenes might be converted to substances with solid tumor activity by the simple expedient of preparing angelate ester and/or glycoside derivatives. By this means, the transport properties might be greatly improved, and the potential evidenced by sesquiterpene lactones in terms of cancer chemotherapeutic agents might then be realized. At the very least, investigations of such sesquiterpenes have been and will continue to be of great academic interest. The structural complexities offer a great challenge and an opportunity for the further development of spectral techniques ranging from mass spectrometry to nuclear magnetic resonance[157] (including use of the nuclear Overhauser effect, NOE) to X-ray crystallographic analyses. At the same time, contributions are being made in this area to botany, chemical taxonomy, and phytochemistry in general.

The diterpenoids constitute the next most frequently encountered group of higher plant antineoplastic agents. In general, the diterpenoids are well known for their wide range of

303

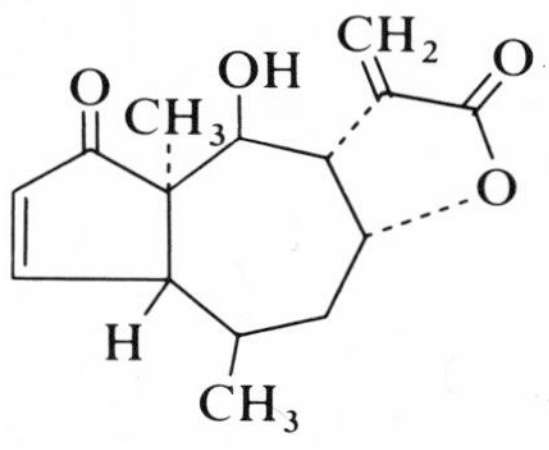

56

Helenalin

PS T/C 220 (3 mg/kg)

312

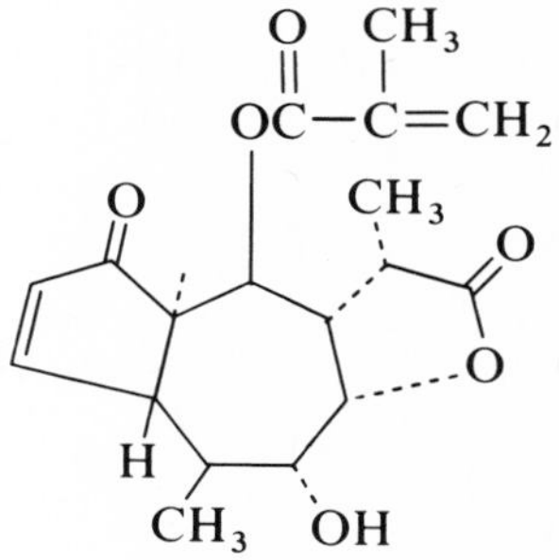

57

Radiatin

PS T/C 161 (25 mg/kg)

312

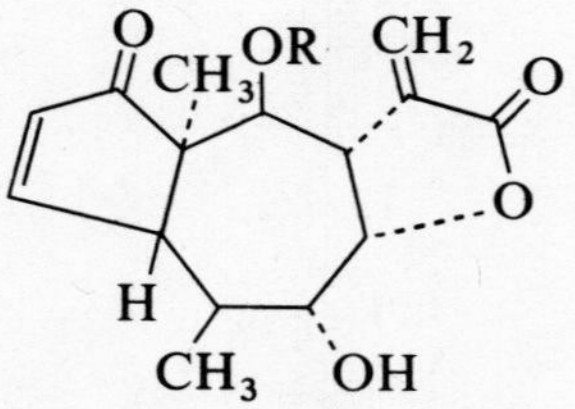

58, R = COCH=C(CH$_3$)$_2$

Fastigilin C

PS T/C 150 (3 mg/kg)

298

$$\overset{\text{CH}_3}{\underset{|}{}}$$

59, R = COC=CHCH$_3$

Multigilin

PS active

157

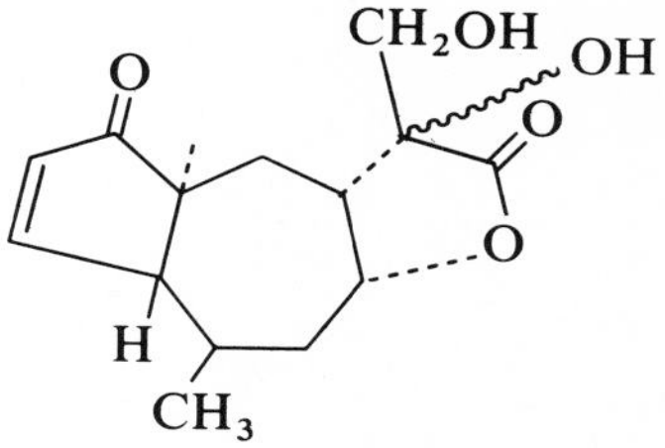

60

Hymenoflorin

LE active

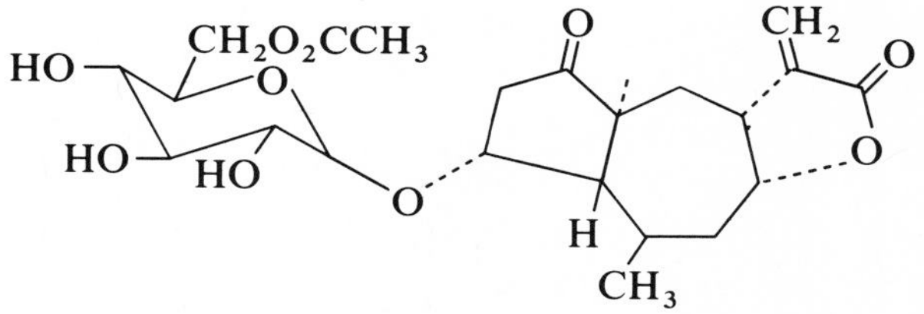

61

Paucin

PS active

biological activity, which includes antibiotic properties and plant growth regulation, such as exhibited by the gibberelin plant hormones. Formation of the major structural classes found among the diterpenes appears to involve appropriate cyclizations of the C_{20} alcohol geranylgeraniol pyrophosphate.[130] The PS active jatrophone[230] represents a very unusual type of macrocyclic diterpene. Kupchan and colleagues found jatrophone (**62**) to be the cytotoxic constituent of *Jatropha gossy piifolia* L. (Euphorbiaceae), a plant with a long history of application for cancer treatment in primitive medicine.[141]

The abietadiene-type tricyclic diterpenes are believed to result from the pyrophosphate ester of geranyl-geraniol functioning as a leaving group in a complete cyclization sequence. Two such abietanes, taxodione (**63**) and taxodone (**64**), isolated from a *Taxodiaceae* species have been found to exhibit some WM activity. Podolide (**65**) represents a diterpene of more complex biogenetic origin. Such norditerpenoid lactones have been found in both the higher and the lower (fungi) plants, but podolide, from the *Taxaceae* species *Protocarpus gracilior* Pilg., was the first located with solid tumor (PS) activity.[204] Interestingly the podolactones A and B are powerful inhibitors of plant cell expansion and division.[131]

The triepoxides **66** and **67** are even more highly substituted abietane diterpenoids that display a potentially useful level of solid tumor activity.[210] Both were isolated from a plant of the Celastraceae family. The Kupchan group also found the potentially important ansa macrolide maytansine (discussed in Chapter 7) in the same family. The NCI–USDA group, led by Perdue, collected the *Maytenus ovatus* (yielding maytansine) in Ethiopia, and the *Tiptery gium wilfordii*, Hook. F., yielding triptolide (**66**) and tripdiolide (**67**) was collected in Taiwan.

The quassinoid bitter principles represent a group of diterpenes with interesting medicinal potential. Glaucarubin has been known since 1960 to be an effective amoebicide and to have antitumor activity.[88,327] The quassinoids have been isolated from plants of the Simaroubaceae family, whose members have a long history of application in primitive medicine, particularly

230

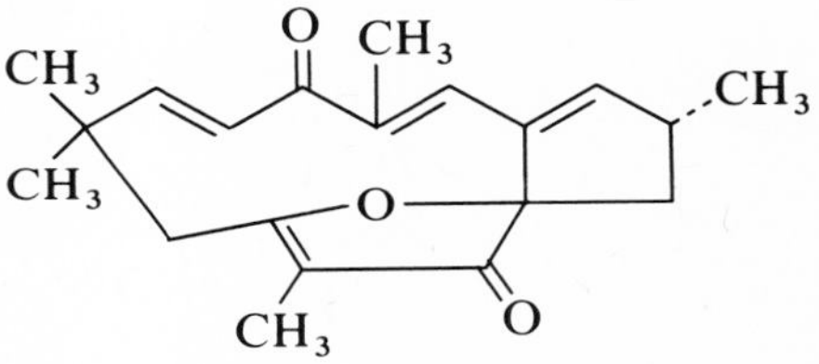

62

Jatrophone

PS active

221

63
Taxodione

WA T/C 36 (25 mg/kg)

221

64
Taxodone

WA T/C 46 (14 mg/kg)

204

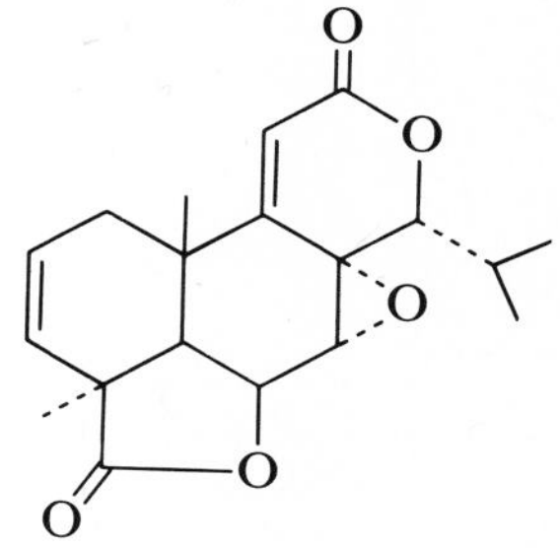

65
Podolide

PS active

210

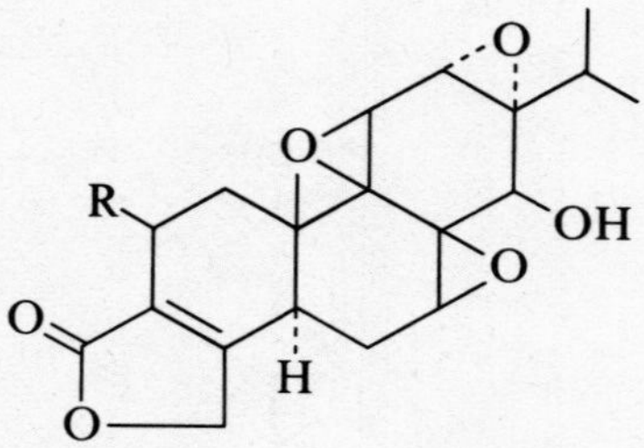

66, R = H

Triptolide

67, R = OH

Tripdiolide

LE active

for their antiamoebic, anti-inflammatory, and antimalarial properties.[327] In 1970, one of these quassinoid constituents, holacanthone (**68**), was reported by the Wall group to inhibit growth of the WA tumor.[416] More recently, Kupchan and co-workers have described the characterization of dehy-droailanthinone (**69**) and bruceantin (**70**).[207] The latter substance displays very good inhibition of the PS leukemia and has sufficient solid tumor activity to warrant consideration for clinical trial in the NCI's programs. Interestingly the bruceantin was isolated from *Brucea antidysenterica* Mill. (Simaroubaceae), an Ethiopian tree with a long history of use in the treatment of cancer.[140]

Cyclization of a macrocyclic diterpenoid precursor can lead to a series of unusual tricyclic diterpenes. One group related to phorbol occurs in species of the plant family Euphorbiaceae.[159] Daphnetoxin (**71**) from *Daphne mezereum*, whose crystal structure was determined by X-ray methods in 1970,[384] provides an illustration. Phorbol derivative **71** is very toxic, and the parent substance (**72**) has been found to be the co-carcinogenic component of *Croton tiglium* L.[68] The seeds of this leafy shrub indigenous to southeast Asia can be expressed or extracted to yield the well-known croton oil. For a man about four seeds and for a horse about 15 seeds represent a lethal dose.[151] More recently, Kupchan and colleagues[232] have isolated and characterized the related diterpenes gniditrin (**73**), gnididin (**74**), and the corresponding cinnamate ester from *Gnidia lamprantha*. These substances have been found to inhibit growth of the PS leukemia.

Another mode of cyclization for a macrocyclic diterpene precursor is that leading to the taxane group. Here taxol (**75**), isolated by the Wall group[423] from stem bark of the western yew, *Taxus brevifolia*, has been found to inhibit growth of the LE, PS, and P-1534 leukemias. Additionally this diterpene (**75**) shows good activity against the WA carcinosarcoma. Consequently taxol has been of interest to the NCI for possible clinical trial. Several other *Taxus* species have also been found to contain taxol.[423]

416

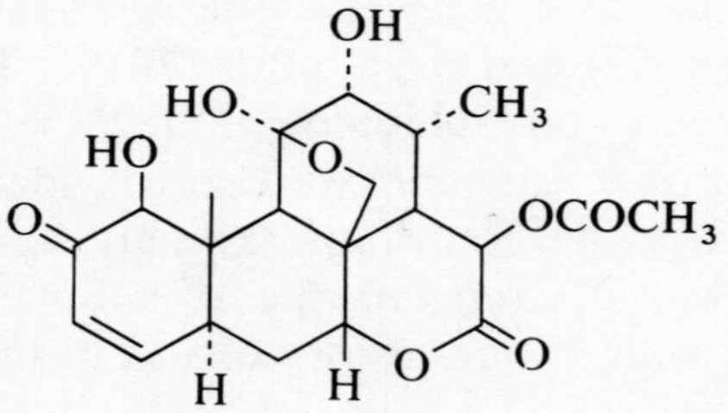

68

Holacanthone

WA active

225

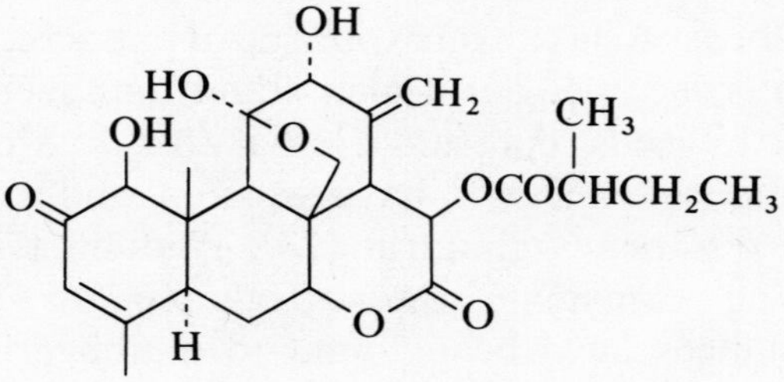

69

Dehydroailanthinone

PS active

207

70

Bruceantin

PS T/C 197

384

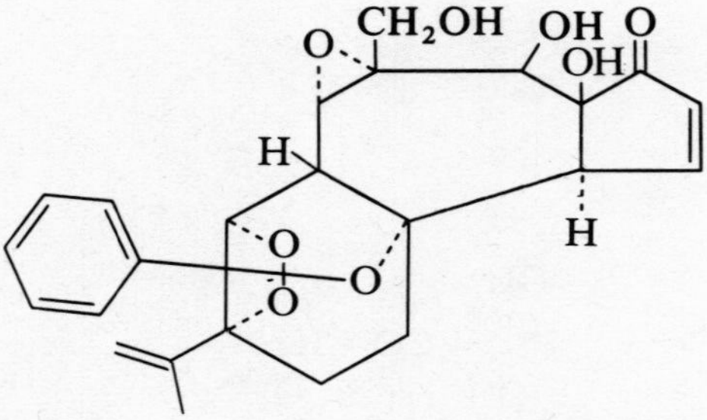

71

Daphnetoxin

LD_{50} $275\,\mu g/kg$

68

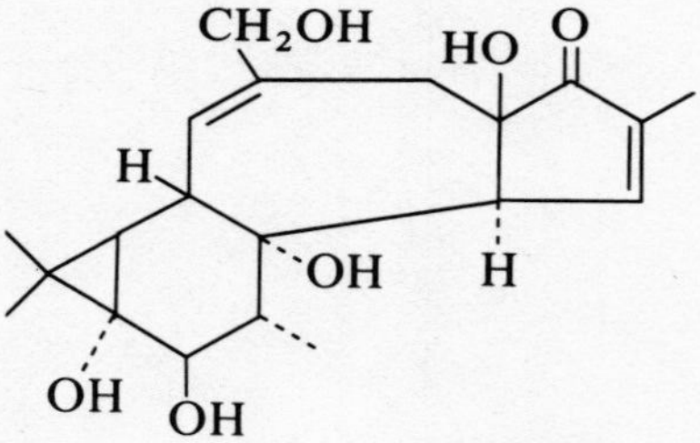

72

Phorbol

Co-carcinogenic

232

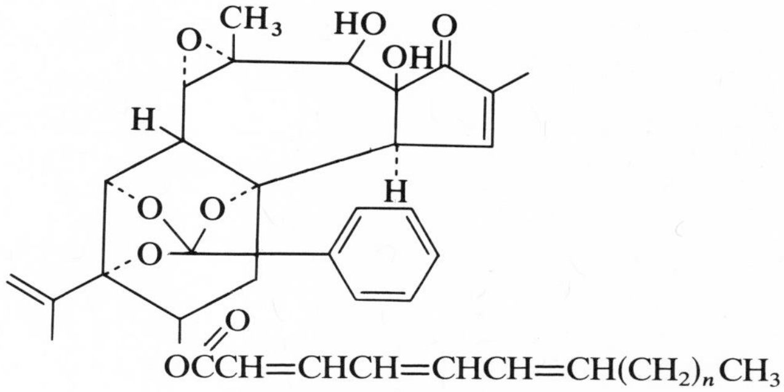

73, Gniditrin ($n = 2$)

74, Gnididin ($n = 4$)

PS active

423

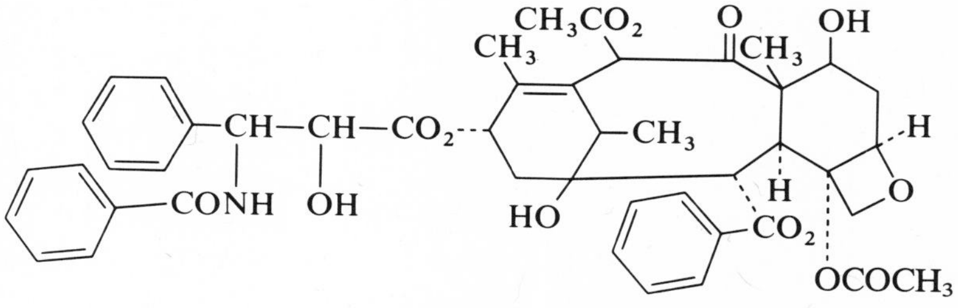

75

Taxol

PS T/C 156

The next class of terpenoids represented in the tabular survey of Volume 2 are two groups of tetracyclic triterpenes. A common pathway for biosynthetic cyclization of the C_{30} hydrocarbon squalene is that leading to lanosterol, an important constituent of mammalian tissue and precursor of the steroidal hormones. The corresponding lanostane carbon skeleton occurs in the sea cucumber saponins, and three of these have recently been found (see Chapter 9) by our group to be cytotoxic agents.

Another group of tetracyclic triterpenes, which apparently arise by a shift of the lanostane 19-methyl group to the 9-position or from a cycloartenol precursor, are the well-known 5α-cucurbitane derivatives.[237] The generally very cytotoxic cucurbitanes are encountered in the Cucurbitaceae family and more recently in the Cruciferae and Scrophulariaceae families. The pronounced toxicity of Cucurbitaceae species was known to ancient peoples and was even recorded in the Bible (Elisha's miracle).[237] Applications (for example, as a purgative) of these cucumber species appear in medical works from the Greek and Roman periods to the British Pharmacopoeia of 1914. The first cucurbitacin (elaterin) was isolated in 1831, and a useful review of this subject has been prepared by Lavie,[237] a long-time contributor to this field. A number of very cytotoxic cucurbitacins have been isolated and characterized by the Lavie and Kupchan[199] groups and studied with respect to antineoplastic activity. Generally the cucurbitacins exhibit a rather narrow therapeutic index, and this has been further substantiated by recent investigations of Konopa and co-workers.[195] However, one would expect that the preparation of suitable derivatives, particularly α,β-unsaturated esters and glycosides, could convert some of these interesting substances into practical drugs for cancer chemotherapy. Some exemplification of this point is provided by the 1972 report of Kupchan and co-workers[229] that datiscoside (**76**) showed inhibitory activity in both the PS and the WM screening systems. In addition, the Lavie group reported antitumor activity for a curcurbitacin glycoside in 1959.[237]

229

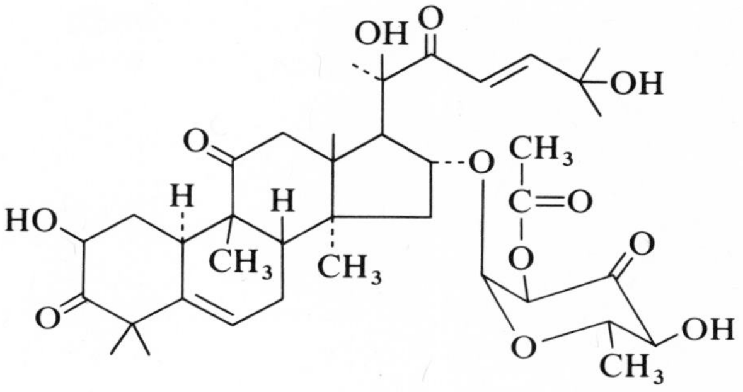

76

Datiscoside

PS and WA active

369

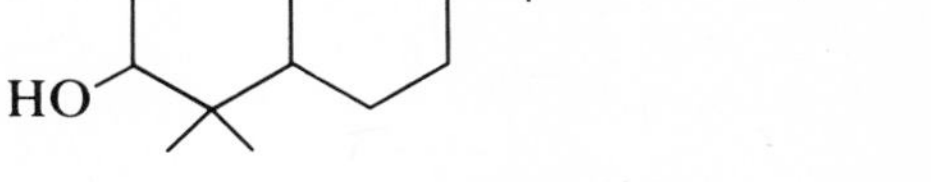

77

Betulin

WA T/C 13 (600 mg/kg)

233

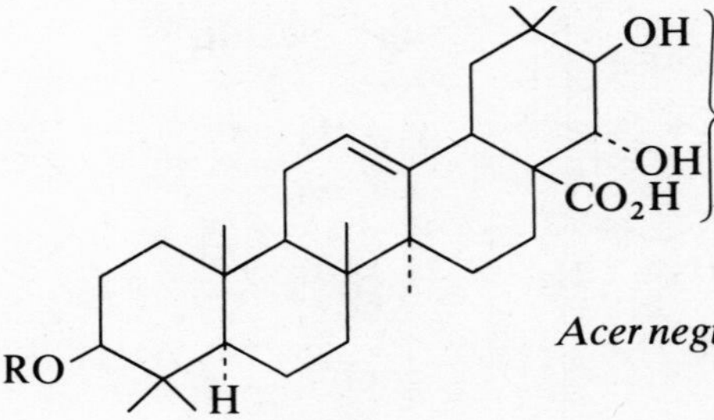

1 : 4 Arabinose, Glucose

Acer negundo L. Saponin P

78, R = $COCH=CHCH=CH_2CH(CH_3)CH_2CH_3$
(all *trans*)

Acerotin

79, R = $-COCH=CHCH=CHCH(CH_3)CH_2CH_3$
(*cis trans*)

Acerocin

S-180 and WA active

Among the pentacyclic triterpenes, the lupane and oleanane derivatives betulin (**77**) and *Acer negundo* L. saponin P. (**78** and **79**) have shown solid tumor activity and are representative of several such related substances. In this respect, betulin (**77**)[306] and the less active lupeol have been isolated from *Alnus oregona* Nutt. (Betulaceae).[232] Betulinic acid has been found by the Cole group[370] to be the active (WA T/C 15 at 500 mg/kg) principal of *Hyptis emoryi* Torr. (Labiatae). Isolation of saponin P from leaves and stems of the Aceraceae species is of more interest because of the level of antineoplastic activity, and this substance has been under consideration as a possible clinical candidate.[231,233] Leaves and stems of the Ethiopian plant *Myrsine africana* L. have yielded a related compound designated myrsine saponin, which has a therapeutic index less promising than that of saponin P.[231] The Farnsworth group[192a] has isolated myrsine saponin from *Wallenia yunquensis* (Urb.) Mez. (Myrsinaceae).

Undoubtedly several of the biosynthetic products mentioned in this chapter will become useful cancer chemotherapeutic agents, and others will inspire synthetic modifications that will in turn yield practical drugs. Even more importantly for the future, there must be a considerable number of even more effective cancer chemotherapeutic drugs yet to be discovered among the more than 200,000 (or 800,000, if a recent estimate of 900,000 plant species is correct) plant species still to be investigated. The same judgment applies to each of those fields of natural products chemistry covered in subsequent chapters.

Chapter 4

Higher Plant Steroids

Further biosynthetic degradation of tetracyclic triterpenes leads to the plant sterols and steroids. The common plant sterols occur ubiquitously, and surprisingly one of the simplest, β-sitosterol (**80**), is known definitely to inhibit growth of the WA neoplasm. Presumably very few of the more highly hydroxylated sterols, such as those functioning as insect hormones and the plant steroids, have been evaluated for antineoplastic activity. This may account in part for the paucity of such substances now known to be antineoplastic agents. Some possible future prospects for the multihydroxylated sterols may be evidenced by the few steroidal saponins, such as digitonin and gitogenin galactoside (**81**), active in the WA system. The latter saponin was found to be an antitumor constituent of *Agave schottii* Engelm. (Amaryllidaceae).[29]

More dependable cytotoxicity and possibly antineoplastic effects can be predicted for multifunctional steroidal lactones; withaferin A (**82**) provides a useful illustration. This interesting withanolide was isolated by Lavie and co-workers from *Withania somniferia* L. Dun. (Solanaceae) and independently, using bioassay techniques, by Kupchan and colleagues.[201] Withaferin A, isolated by the latter investigators from another Solanaceae species (*Acnistus arborescens* L. Schlecht), showed both cytotoxicity and some solid tumor activity against WA. The plant material (leaves) used for this study was collected in Costa

145

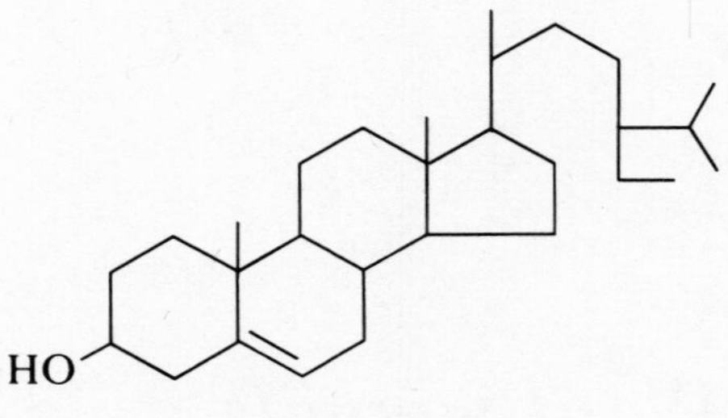

80

β-Sitosterol

WA T/C 3 (29–45 mg/kg)

29

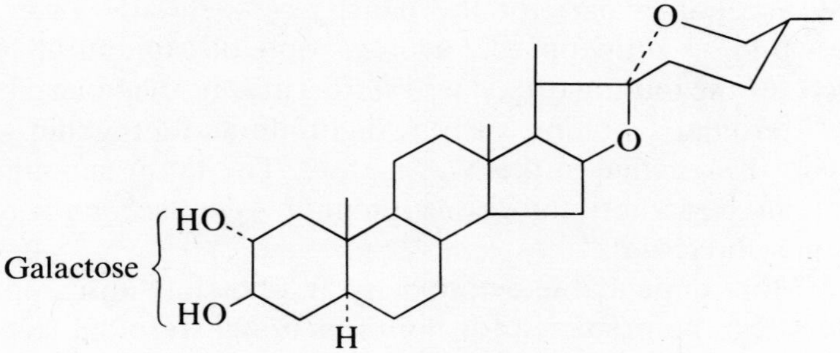

Galactose

81

Gitogenin galactoside

WA T/C 17 (65 mg/kg)

201

82

Withaferin A

WA and S-180 active

Rica and is known to have been employed in primitive treatment of cancer. The list of new withanolides has recently been increased by the addition of Q and R.[193]

The only bufadienolide known to occur in both plants and animals is hellebrigenin (**83**); the 3-acetate derivative **83** was found to be the WA inhibitor of the Ethiopian plant *Bersama abyssinica* Fresen. (Melianthaceae).[217] Subsequently a total of four new cytotoxic (KB) bufadienolides were isolated from the same plant.[217,228] In 1957, our group began a long-term study of bufadienolides as potential antineoplastic agents. Pertinent aspects of these studies are reviewed in Chapter 10 in connection with the amphibian venoms. As part of this study, the plant bufadienolide proscillaridin A (**84**) was subjected to cytotoxicity and anticancer evaluation. While this substance displays substantial KB cytotoxicity, it has not proved of any interest in the *in vivo* systems, such as LE, PS, BI and LL.[180,298] At the same time, synthesis of a suitable derivative of glycoside **84** or the aglycone scillarenin (**85**)[180] has been attempted where the cytotoxicity might be translated to *in vivo* antineoplastic properties. Proscillaridin A is now employed in medicine for certain types of heart failure and is still obtained from the Mediterranean plant *Scilla maritima*. Interestingly this plant has been used from approximately 3500 B.C. for its diuretic and heart effects. The ancient Egyptians were so impressed by the physiological potency of *Scilla maritima* extracts that they erected a temple in its honor.[307]

Several of the naturally occurring cardenolide glycosides, such as digitoxin, are well known for their medical utility in maintaining heart rhythm. These cardiac glycosides have a very specific effect on the transport of sodium and potassium ions across cell membranes. The mechanism by which sodium and potassium are transported against the electrochemical gradient of the cell membrane is based on a membrane-bound adenosine triphosphatase that needs magnesium ions and is activated by changes in the concentrations of potassium and sodium ions. The enzyme involved is generally referred to as Na^+, K^+-ATPase and is specifically inhibited by the cardenolides. The same

217

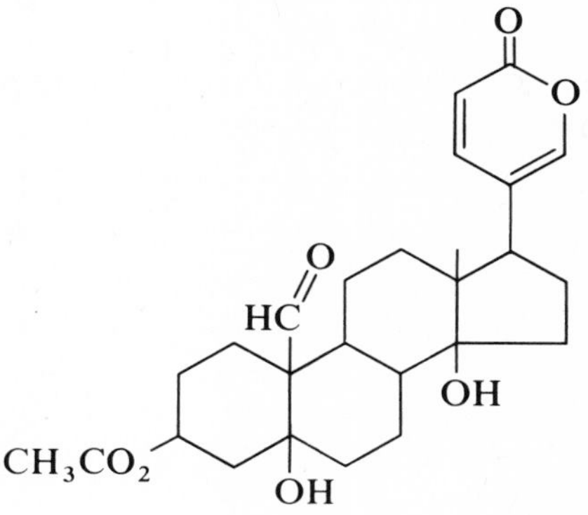

83

Hellebrigenin 3-acetate

WA T/C 25 (8 mg/kg)
KB ED_{50} 0.28 μg/ml

180

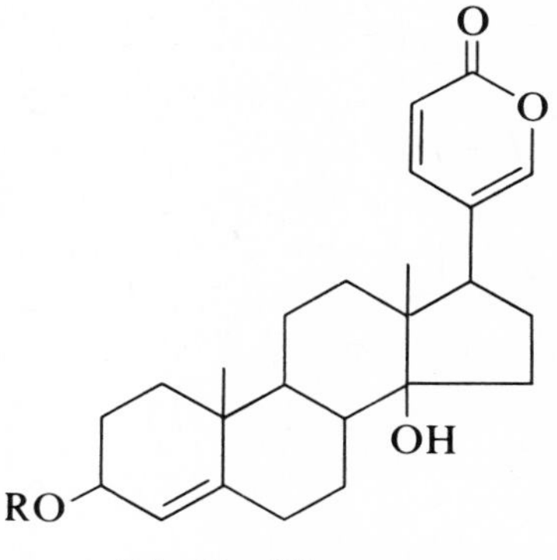

84, R = Rhamnose

Proscillaridin A

KB ED_{50} 2.6 × 10^{-7} μg/ml

85, R = H

Scillarenin

182
188

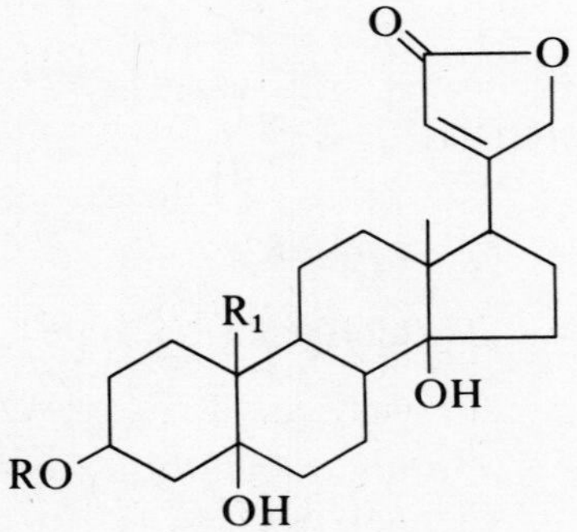

86, R = L-Rhamnose, R$_1$ = —CHO

Convallatoxin

KB ED$_{50}$ 2×10^{-3} μg/ml

87, R = H, R$_1$ = —CH$_3$

Periplogenin

enzyme seems to be involved in the transport of amino acids, sugars, amines, and *p*-amino-hippuric acid across cell membranes. Members of both the bufadienolide and cardenolide classes of steroids display this very specific inhibitory effect on the enzyme, with resultant effects on heart muscle contractility.[398]

Kupchan[217] has suggested that the anticancer action of hellebrigenin 3-acetate (**83**) may be due in part to the inhibition of amino acid accumulation by neoplastic cells. For similar reasons, we expect that either suitable bufadienolides and cardenolides will be isolated and found to possess useful antineoplastic activity and/or they will be obtained by synthetic manipulations of biosynthetic products. To date, the small number of cardenolides evaluated have been found to display pronounced cytotoxicity (KB) but have not shown *in vivo* anticancer properties. The very cytotoxic convallatoxin (**86**) from the bulbs of *Ornithogalum umbellatum* provides an example in terms of KB cell line growth inhibition.[188] However, this cardiac glycoside and many other known substances of this type have probably never been adequately evaluated against experimental *in vivo* tumor systems. In order to make such substances more readily available for biological evaluation, we have been developing total syntheses in this area. A recently completed route to periplogenin (**87**) provides an example.[182] In short, the bufadienolides, cardenolides, and withanolides present interesting leads in need of extended exploration and development.

Chapter 5

Higher Plant Lignans

Plant species of the Berberidaceae family, particularly from the *Berberis* and *Epimedium* genera, have been used in the treatment of warts and various solid tumors in China and India from at least the second century A.D.[145] Another member of this family, *Podophyllum peltatum* L., commonly known as the may apple or mandrake, has been used for similar purposes in the United States from at least the 18th century. Perhaps the earliest use of this plant was by the Penobscot Indians of Maine. The alcohol-soluble portion from the dried roots and rhizomes is known as podophyllum, a material that appeared in the U.S. Pharmacopeia from 1820 to 1942.[301]

    The best-established human neoplastic diseases of viral origin are the various warts.[332] Podophyllum was used by the early settlers of Louisiana and Missouri to treat the venereal wart condyloma acuminatum. Later, when podophyllum was given an early clinical evaluation, it was found to cause complete regression of such warts, and by local application in the female urethra it was shown to cause regression of soft papillomas.[146] The podophyllin resin was also found useful in the treatment of verruca vulgaris and to have a local cytostatic effect as early as 1861.[24] A year earlier, podophyllotoxin (**88**) was isolated from the resin, and a nearly complete structure was proposed by Späth in 1933. The chemistry and antineoplastic activity of podophyllin constituents was under active investigation by

97

Hartwell in the 1940's at the National Cancer Institute. An excellent review of the history, chemistry, and pharmacology of podophyllum to about 1957 has been prepared by Hartwell and Schrecker.[147]

In 1947, Hartwell reported the inhibition of sarcoma 37 by podophyllotoxin, and subsequently this ligand (usually formed in the plant by dimerization of cinnamyl alcohols at the α-positions) was found capable of similar activity with several other transplantable tumor systems and of arresting cell division in metaphase.[146,374] Later podophyllotoxin (**88**) was given a limited clinical trial, but because of poor solubility characteristics and a low therapeutic index, these clinical investigations were discontinued. Related lignan constituents of podophyllin, including the α- and β-peltatins,[412] proved active but seemingly did not offer better clinical promise. More recently, a series of related lignans, including desoxypodophyllotoxin (**89**), have been isolated from the Japanese evergreen tree *Thujopsis dolabrata* (L. fil.) Sieb. and Zucc. (Cupressaceae).[4] The 3'-desmethyl derivative (**90**) of podophyllotoxin has been isolated by Farnsworth and colleagues[430] along with podophyllotoxin and the peltatins from *Linum album* (Linaceae). Two (**91** and **92**) members of the very rare bisbenzocyclooctadiene lignan type were found by the Kupchan group[208] to be PS active constituents of *Steganotaenia araliacea* Hochst. In time, it will be interesting to compare the antineoplastic evaluation of steganangin (**92**), an angelate ester, with the more frequently encountered podophyllotoxin-type lignans and with the angelate esters of sesquiterpene lactones. The total synthesis of ($\pm$)-steganacin was achieved early in 1976 by the Kende group.[190]

Fortunately the promise of podophyllotoxin-type lignans did not go unnoticed, and beginning in the 1950's, efforts by a small number of groups[3,375,301] was directed at synthetic modifications that might prove more effective clinically. Similar efforts continued in the 1960's and two 4'-demethyl-epipodophyllotoxin glucosides (**93** and **94**) now supplied by Sandoz, Ltd. (Basel) give evidence of being clinically useful

146

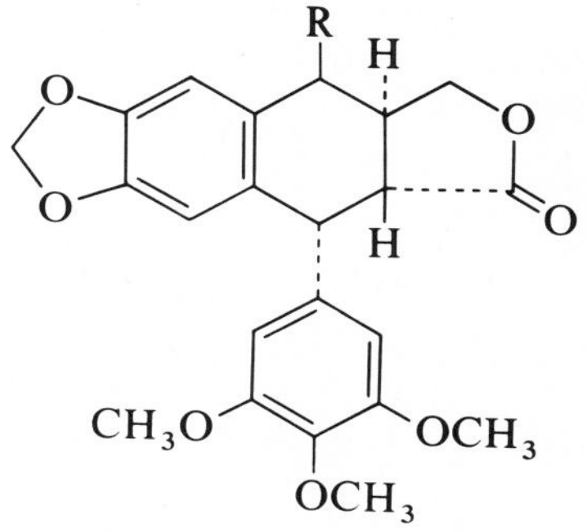

88, R = OH

Podophyllotoxin

PS T/C 171, WA T/C 27

89, R = H

Desoxypodophyllotoxin

PS T/C 148

430

90

3′-Desmethylpodophyllotoxin

PS T/C 130

208

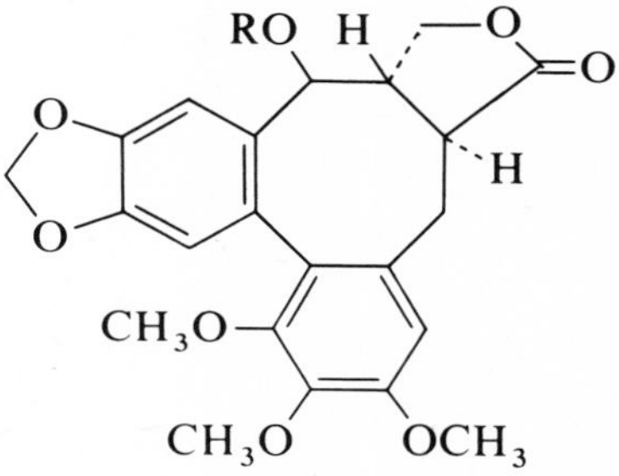

91, R = —COCH$_3$

Steganacin

92, R = —CO

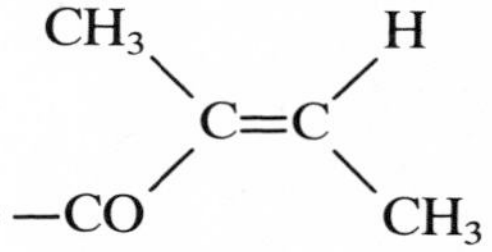

Steganangin

PS active

434

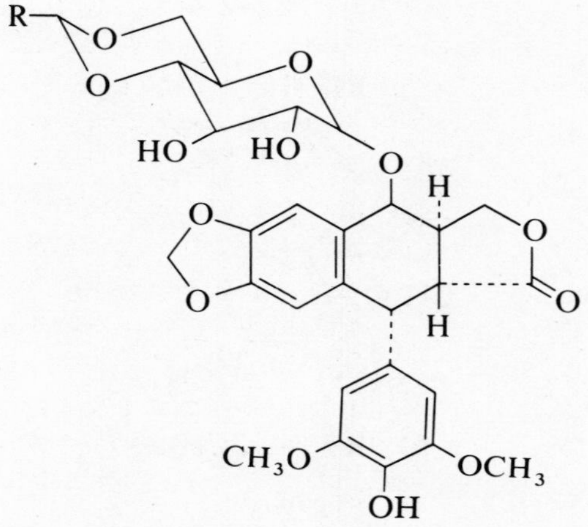

93, R = —CH₃

NSC 141540 (VP-16-213)
    LE T/C 250, PS T/C 241, B1 T/C 280
    WA, S-180, P-1534 active

94, R = (thiophene)

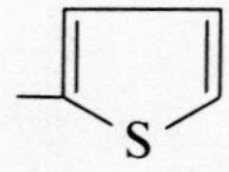

NSC 122819 (VM-26)
    LE T/C 300, PS T/C 250
    WA, P-815 active

cancer chemotherapeutic drugs.[281,378] Both of these podophyllotoxin derivatives, unlike the parent substance, show a pronounced antineoplastic effect in the murine LE screening system.[280,374] Of particular importance is the dramatic activity of 4′-demethylepipodophyllotoxin 9-(4,6-O-thenylidene)-β-D-glucopyranoside (**94**) against intracerebral LE. Mice given an intracerebral dose of 10^4 LE cells and intraperitoneal injections of glycoside **94** had a 150% increase in medial survival. Glucosides **93** and **94** are both even more effective against the L1210 leukemia transplanted by the intraperitoneal route.

The most exciting recent application of epipodophyllotoxin derivative **94** has been in the treatment of human intracranial neoplasms by the Walker clinical group.[374] In an expert clinical study of acetal **94**, Walker found a 38% overall remission rate in patients displaying clinically measurable neoplastic disease. The remission rate included two of nine patients with malignant gliomas and, at the time of writing, a more than 15-month progression-free interval for the responding patients. The study was conducted on patients with an inoperable intracranial cancer or with an incompletely removed malignant neoplasm. The management and cure of brain and other central nervous system cancer by chemotherapy are very urgently needed. Hopefully, with the future use of acetal **94** in combination with other drugs crossing the blood–brain barrier, such as the nitrosoureas, this most worthwhile goal will be realized.

One of the first studies of podophyllotoxin derivative **94** in combination with natulan and prednisolone for Hodgkin's therapy has been completed. An 84% total of partial and complete remission was noted. In the resistant group, 75% presented Hodgkin's sarcoma upon postmortem examination.[93]

The use of the very closely related acetaldehyde acetal **93** in the treatment of 11 patients with oat cell carcinoma of the lung resulted in 8 responses. Four out of six patients with ovarian cancer responded.[179] While acetal **93** is less active in experimental tumor systems than the thiophene aldehyde acetal **94**, it does have a larger therapeutic index and offers the possibility of eventually being useful by oral administration instead of the present IV route for both acetals.

A reading of this chapter should leave little doubt that given the necessary talent, time, and resources, very useful clinical drugs can be prepared by appropriate synthetic modifications of the original biosynthetic product. One frequently encounters the rather pessimistic view that the first active substance discovered is usually the best, but this is far from the truth and there is ample evidence to the contrary. Eventually even more effective podophyllotoxin derivatives will be discovered in living organisms and/or obtained by synthetic procedures. Current successes in the lignan field with synthetic modification should serve as a very useful guide for further developing the terpenoid and steroid leads outlined in Chapters 3 and 4.

Chapter 6

Quinones, Flavans, and Other Nonnitrogenous Higher Plant Products

All of the miscellaneous plant products ranging from hydrocarbons to the highly oxygenated polysaccharides have been grouped into this chapter. In general they have shown only marginal cytotoxic and/or *in vivo* antitumor properties. The gallic acid that we found to be the cytotoxic constituent of two Utah plants, *Rhus trilobata* (Anacardiaceae) and *Oenothera caespitosa* (Onagraceae), seems to be the smallest molecular-weight natural product so far isolated with those properties.[323] A substance of comparable size with *in vivo* anticancer activity is crotepoxide (**95**), reported by Kupchan[218] to be the antineoplastic agent of *Croton macrostachys* Hochst. *ex.* A. Rich (Euphorbiaceae). Cyclohexane diepoxide **95** was found to have activity against the LL system at a toxic dose and also to show inhibition of the WM tumor system. From a biogenetic viewpoint, crotepoxide seems related to shikimic acid. Ichihara and co-workers[288] have completed a total synthesis of (±) crotepoxide.

Among the aromatic hydrocarbon derivatives, very few have given evidence of *in vivo* antineoplastic action and that only of a low order. Two such examples are aristolochic acid (**96**)

218

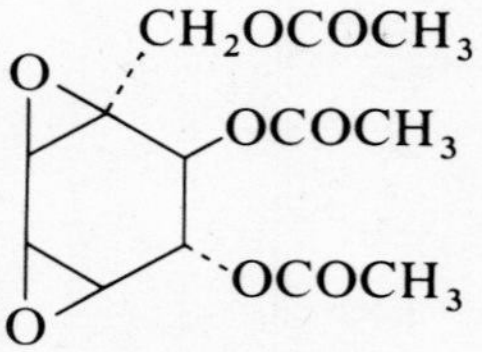

95

Crotepoxide

WA T/C 22 (450 mg/kg)

213

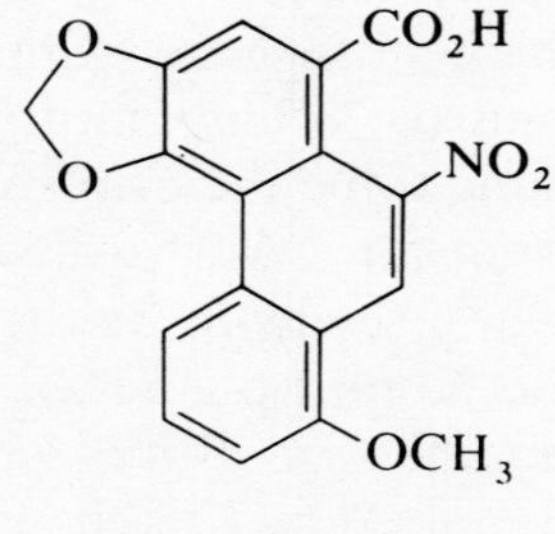

96

Aristolochic acid

CA 755 active

61
313

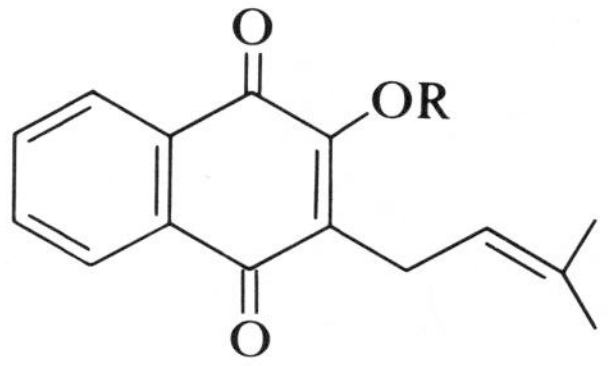

97, R = H

Lapachol

WA T/C 27

R =

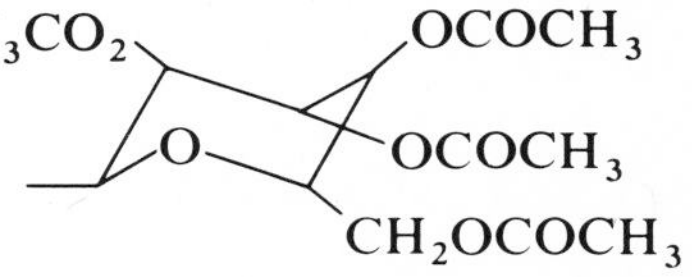

98

PS T/C 180

from *Aristolochia indica*[213] (Aristolochiaceae) and lapachol (**97**) from the heartwood of several *Tabeluia* species (e.g., Araliaceae) *Bignoniaceae Tectona grandis* L. Fil. (Verbenaceae).[61,145,313,356] Lapachol (**97**) has a long and interesting history, beginning with its isolation and structural determination by the gifted experimentalist Hooker at the end of the 19th century. Also lapachol served as a starting point for the development of antimalarial drugs during World War II by Fieser and co-workers.[99] More recently a phase I clinical trial of lapachol was begun but not brought to a definite conclusion.[33,334] Meanwhile quinone **97** has been produced commercially in Brazil for the clinical management of cancer. When available, the results of these trials will surely be of interest.[61] In the hope that lapachol might prove useful, we completed a practical total synthesis of this compound in 1967.[313] Meanwhile a Brazilian group has prepared the tetraacetyl glucose derivative **98** and found it to exhibit pronounced PS activity in contrast to lapachol, which is inactive in that screening system.[61] Quite possibly the glycoside (**98**) derivative of lapachol has better transport properties *in vivo* and may eventually prove to be useful clinically.

From a structure activity standpoint, it is noteworthy that the unprotected glucoside derivative of lapachol did not display the PS inhibition shown by the corresponding tetraacetate **98**. Consequently partial and/or completely esterified glycosides may be an important structural feature for synthetic modification of some naturally occurring antineoplastic agents. Such structural manipulations might be of interest with some of the otherwise only cytotoxic flavin derivatives[413] recorded in the tables of Volume 2.

Chapter 7

Higher Plant Alkaloids, Amides, and Ansa Macrolides

A majority of the biosynthetic products with substantial activity against solid neoplastic disease contain one or more basic or nearly neutral nitrogen atoms. About 15 of these compounds are either now in clinical trial as cancer chemotherapeutic drugs or are being considered for such application. The discussion of this section will be centered primarily on these promising candidates for cancer treatment. A comparable number of nitrogen-containing anticancer agents (usually classed as antitumor antibiotics) from the lower plants will be found in the following chapter dealing with microorganism biosynthetic products.

Most of the nitrogen-containing plant antineoplastic constituents have *in vivo* activity as well as cytotoxic effects detectable by the KB screen. A majority can be classed as alkaloids. Some highlights resulting from this early area of endeavor will be discussed first. Strictly speaking, alkaloids are physiologically and optically active plant products containing a basic nitrogen atom. These substances were first classified as vegetable alkali, and their systematic chemical investigation was already under way in 1812. The term *alkaloid* ("alkalilike") for the nitrogenous bases of plants was suggested by the pharmacist Meissner in 1819.[294] Early investigations of alkaloids were restricted to relatively few plant families, such as the Rubiaceae (cinchona, ipecac), Papaveraceae (the poppies, aporphines), Solanaceae (deadly nightshade, potato, tobacco), Papilionaceae (lupines), Berberidaceae (bisbenzylisoquinoline), Menispermaceae (bis-benzylisoquinoline), Ranunculaceae (delphinine), Rutaceae (acridines, furoquinolines), and Apocynaceae (dogbane, queb-racho, yohimbine). The number of such families has increased from about 40, 25 years ago, to a much greater number today.

A comprehensive picture of alkaloid distribution in plants can be obtained from the results of a recent study by the Farnsworth group[377] in which extracts from 4,888 plant species from the National Cancer Institute (NCI) collection were pro-vided by Hartwell for alkaloid screening. Of these various plant species, 1,336 gave positive alkaloid reactions. In the most recent addition to this survey, 1,005 plant extracts gave 190 (18.9%) positive alkaloid tests. Of these, 153 species were previously unknown to contain alkaloids.[377] In a similar exten-sive survey, 3,700 species of New Guinea plants were screened for alkaloids. Of some 2,000 species tested with Meyer's reag-ent, about 10% seemed to contain alkaloids.[138] Thus the alkaloids so far isolated probably account for less than 1% of those remaining to be discovered, and their distribution in the plant kingdom will turn out to be quite broad.

While the alkaloids with substantial *in vivo* antineoplastic properties were being selected and correlated for special emphasis, some structure/activity relationships became appar-ent. The intercalative binding to DNA of the type attributed to ellipticine may well be operative, at least in part, with several other aromatic and therefore planar compounds. Several appear to fit the N–O–O-triangulation hypothesis suggested by Zee–Cheng and Cheng in 1970.[438] This empirical relationship (**99**) based on closely defined interatomic distances and a trian-gular relationship between a nitrogen and two oxygen atoms may suggest the proper orientation of such atoms for useful transport properties. The triangulation concept seems to fit camptothecin, vincristine, methotrexate, cytosine arabinoside, several of the anthracycline anticancer antibiotics (such as daunomycin, included in the next chapter), and several other types of known anticancer agents. Since these compounds are believed to owe their antineoplastic properties to a variety of biochemical mechanisms, the specific spacial arrangement of three such electronegative atoms may simply be a useful feature for proper transport. Other structural features have occurred to this reviewer, and some of these have been employed in the grouping of the alkaloids and alkaloidlike compounds that follow. A very impressive characteristic of the first group to be considered is the pyrrolizidine ring (**100**, $n = 1$) or a homologue (**100**, $n = 2$ or 3). The pyrrolizidine ring system characteristic of the *Senecio* alkaloids was unknown until the first structural determination was completed.[240] This bridgehead-type nitrogen arrangement appears consistently in the first grouping of alkaloids to be considered, namely, **101–108**.

The genus *Senecio* is the largest of the Compositae family and includes over 1,000 species. Many of these species are known to contain alkaloids bearing the pyrrolizidine ring system. Some plants of the Leguminosae (*Crotalaria* genus) and Boraginaceae (for example, *Heliotropium* genus) families contain related alkaloids. The NCI's arrangement with the Australian CSIRO group of Culvenor and colleagues[69] eventually led to the current interest in indicine *N*-oxide (**101**). The principal alkaloid in extracts of *Heliotropium indicum* has been found by Mattocks[259] to be indisine (obtained after reduction of the *N*-oxide). *Senecio* alkaloid **101** exhibits a potentially useful level and spectrum of antitumor activity, and if the hepatotoxicity generally associated with this type of alkaloid proves manageable, it may become of further interest.

The *Senecio* alkaloids have a long history of being responsible for chronic liver disease—for example, in livestock—and the substances responsible have been shown to exert an irreversible antimitotic action on liver cells, leading to megalocytosis (enlarged cells). These alkaloids are also known to be mutagenic and cause chromosome breakage. Generally the hepatotoxicity seems correlatable with reduced base strength and reduced water solubility.[69] The same physical properties, including water-lipid partition coefficients, can be correlated with

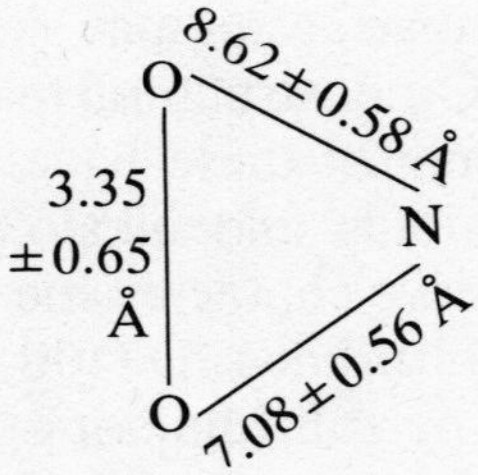

$$8.62 \pm 0.58 \text{ Å}$$

O

$$3.35 \pm 0.65 \text{ Å}$$

N

O $7.08 \pm 0.56 \text{ Å}$

99

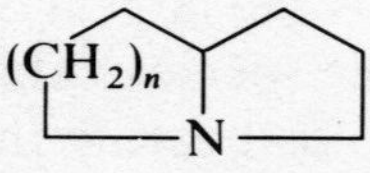

$(CH_2)_n$ N

100

259

HO CH$_2$OC—C—CHCH$_3$

OH OH

N

O

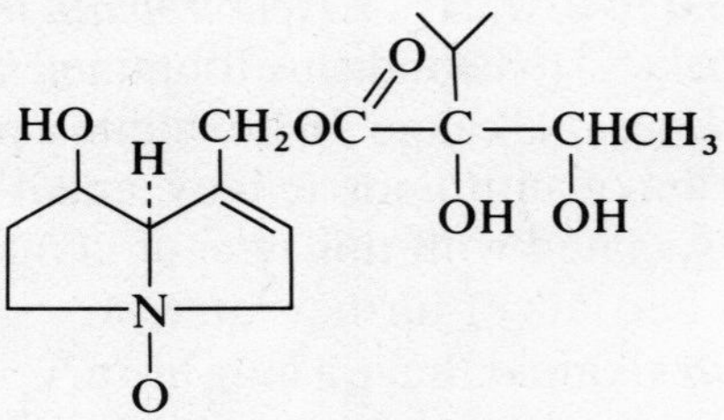

101

Indicine *N-oxide*

LE T/C 140, PS T/C 200, B1 T/C 153

antineoplastic activity. If the appropriate structural modifications can be made, a derivative might be obtained with selective action on hepatomas.

The Asclepiadaceae family is probably better known for its cardenolide constituents, but this group of over 700 species (and over 320 genera) does produce a small number of species with alkaloids. The Australian slender vine *Tylophora crebriflora* and a plant from the Moraceae family, *Ficus septica*, are both known to produce the phenanthroindolizidine alkaloid tylocrebrine (**102**).[123] The isolation, characterization, and synthesis of this alkaloid was reported by Gellert and co-workers[111] in 1962. This was followed 2 years later by a summary of the inhibitory effects of tylocrebrine against LE.

The quinoline alkaloid camptothecin (**103**), originally isolated in 1966 by the Wall group[417] from the Chinese tree *Camptotheca acuminata* (Nyssaceae), was the focal point of intense interest by the NCI for several years. Because of preliminary indications of activity against colon cancer during a phase I clinical trial, the need for a convenient source of camptothecin intensified. The supply of stem wood from the few ornamental *Camptotheca* trees in private collections in the United States was rapidly exhausted, and the U.S. Department of Agriculture (USDA) undertook cultivation of this plant in California. At the same time it was hoped that total synthesis could provide more immediate needs, and a number of very skillful chemical groups accepted the challenge. To date, 10 novel syntheses have been completed and 9 of these have been summarized by Shamma and Georgiev,[368] who successfully completed one of the routes. Just recently, Corey and co-workers[65] completed a total synthesis of the natural 20(S)-camptothecin (**103**).

Unfortunately a phase II clinical trial of comptothecin against gastrointestinal cancer was not particularly encouraging.[271] Since camptothecin has a very good spectrum of activity against experimental tumor systems and is known to interfere[244] with progression of S or early G_2 cells into mitosis, pyridine **103** may still have a future clinically. As mentioned in Chapter 2,

111
145

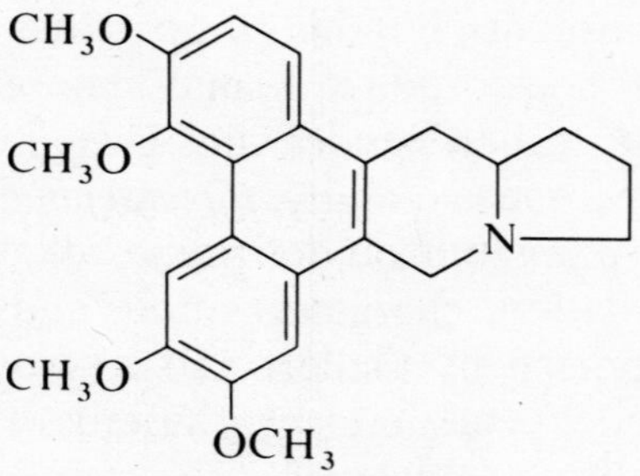

102

Tylocrebrine

LE T/C 168 (10 mg/kg)
PS T/C 170, WA T/C 41

417

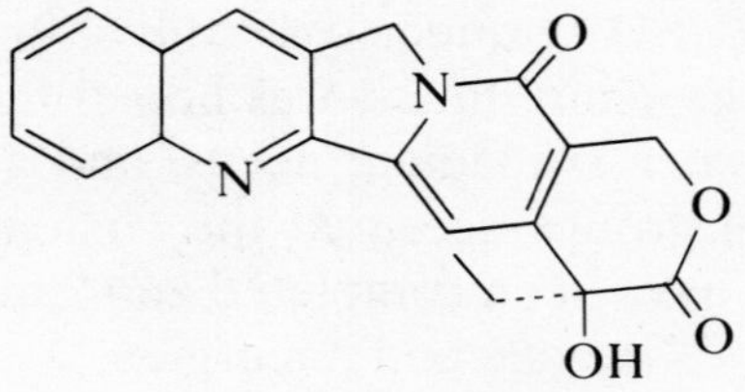

103

Camptothecin

LE T/C 200 (0.25–1 mg/kg)
WA T/C 0

organic chemical, pharmacological, and clinical groups in the People's Republic of China have camptothecin in clinical trial, and this expanded study may prove quite fruitful. At the same time, the Chinese investigators[299] have the 10-hydroxy- and 10-methoxy-camptothecins[424a] under study. Both of the latter compounds show promising anticancer activity in several animal tumor systems. The extensive structural modifications of camptothecin have been another area of substantial interest,[322,368] and hopefully some of these endeavors will lead to clinically useful drugs. Overall camptothecin is an attractive substance for further study. Camptothecin seems to have most of the structural attributes, including potential for an α,β-unsaturated lactone and nearly planar structure, likely to confer antineoplastic activity.

The *Vinca* alkaloids vincristine (**104**) and vinblastine (**105**) have already been successfully introduced into clinical practice as cancer chemotherapeutic drugs. Both have been isolated from leaves of the white-flowered periwinkle *Vinca rosea*, a member of the usually tropical and woody Apocynaceae family. The *Vinca* genus is native to southern Europe and the Middle East, while the closely related *Catharanthus* genus is native to Madagascar and India. Because some of these species, such as *Vinca rosea*, make attractive ornamentals, they now have a wide distribution.

The potential of *Vinca rosea* components in cancer chemotherapy was discovered by Noble and colleagues at the University of Western Ontario.[282] This very important discovery had origins beginning in 1949 and makes a nice illustration of how careful scientific observation and judgment is crucial to progress. A tea made from *Vinca rosea* leaves had been used in Jamaica for treatment of diabetes mellitus. Samples of the plant were forwarded to Noble for study. Neither extracts from the Jamaican *Vinca rosea* nor similar extracts marketed in England for supposed treatment of diabetes seemed to alter the blood sugar of experimental animals. Consequently, instead of continued oral use of the extract, it was given by the intravenous route to rats. The result was quite unexpected: the animals died

277
386
387
434

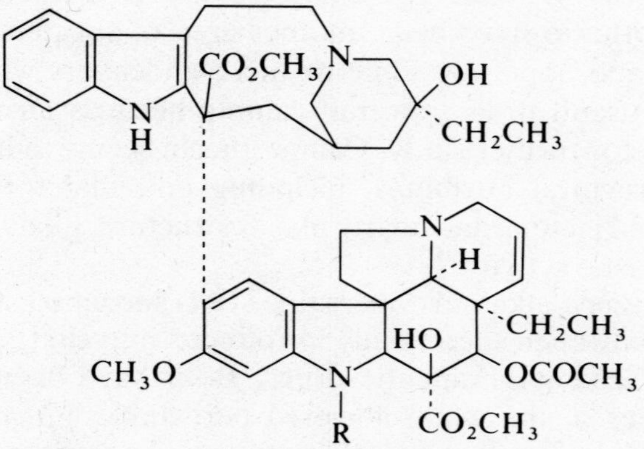

104, R = —CHO

Vincristine

LE T/C 147, PS T/C 242, B1 T/C 189

105, R = —CH₃

Vinblastine

LE T/C 140, PS T/C 212, B1 T/C 220

in 5–7 days. Upon autopsy, the rats showed multiple abscesses resulting from septicemia, particularly in the liver and kidneys. A subsequent culture confirmed *Pseudomonas* spp., and it seemed that some components of the extract might have been immunosuppressive. Indeed the extract was found to cause a rapid drop in the white blood count, bone marrow depression, and granulocytopenia. By 1955, the Noble group had begun a detailed chemical study of *Vinca rosea* with the prospect of isolating the component(s) that might have application in leukemia. The actual isolation work was guided by bioassay and would seem to be one of the first such applications in cancer chemotherapy. Soon the new alkaloid vincaleukoblastine, now known as vinblastine, was isolated and found to produce severe leukopenia in rats.[282] Meanwhile Svoboda and Johnson at the Lilly Research Laboratories found that *Vinca rosea* fractions were active against the P-1534 acute lymphocytic leukemia, and vincristine was isolated.[173,174,175,277]

Indole alkaloids **104** and **105** have since been found to inhibit the cell cycle at metaphase. Higher dose vincristine is inhibitory in S phase and vinblastine in both S and late G_1.[64,253] As already mentioned in Chapters 1 and 2, both compound **104** and compound **105** are now in clinical use.[359] In addition to the application of vincristine in the NCI's MOPP treatment for Hodgkin's disease, vinblastine as a single-agent treatment for monocytic leukemia has recently led to a 60% remission rate.[110] The dose-limiting factor of vincristine is its neurologic toxicity, which is rather unusual among cancer chemotherapeutic drugs.[429] Although both vincristine and vinblastine, along with procarbazine, are known to be teratogens in animals, the few cases involving human pregnancies so far known have resulted in the delivery of normal infants. A recent study using 3H-vincristine with murine leukemia cells *in vitro* has suggested that drug resistance may be due at least in part to impaired accumulation and binding of vincristine within the cell.[32] The nearly identical alkaloids **104** and **105** have in the aspidospermidine unit a bridgehead nitrogen that may again be important for activity. The excellent chemical investigation of such *Vinca* alkaloids[394] by Kutney at the University of British Columbia should lead to a much better understanding of structure/activity relationships in this series and to the first total synthesis.[234] Indeed (±)-vindoline (the most prominent alkaloid in *Vinca rosea* L. leaves),[294] the aspidospermine ring system of vincristine and vinblastine, has just been synthesized by the Büchi group.[5]

A joint program (evaluating plants selected by Perdue) between the NCI and the USDA, led by Smith,[329] has resulted in another group of bridgehead-nitrogen–containing alkaloids of substantial promise. Two varieties of *Cephalotaxus harringtonia* gave extracts active against both the PS and the LE murine leukemias. Fractionation and characterization of the active components provided the new cephalotaxine esters **106–108** and an isomer designated isoharringtonine.[266,329] The parent alcohol cephalotaxine amounts to some 50% of the total alkaloids present but is inactive against the rodent tumor systems. Interestingly acetylcephalotaxine is also inactive, and slight changes in the harringtonine-type ester side chain significantly affect the antitumor response (*cf.* **106–108**). The results of a future study aimed at modifying the cephalotaxine ester unit should yield very important information. Obviously the esters are necessary for transport and may provide useful structural leads for improving the efficiency of other biosynthetic products. Harringtonine, for example, has been shown to inhibit the initiation of protein biosynthesis.[164a] In 1972, a total synthesis of cephalotaxine was completed,[14] and in 1975 a rather short-path 8-step total synthesis was reported.[366] Meanwhile a synthesis of the deoxyharringtonine (**107**) ester side chain has been completed.[13] Under the direction of Engle at the NCI the cephalotaxine synthesis is being developed into a practical source of supply.

Currently the harringtonine-type alkaloids are of interest for possible clinical trial in the NCI's programs and are already being considered for such trial in the People's Republic of China.[299] Given the high level of PS response exhibited by ester **106** and related substances, one or more compounds in this series should become clinically useful and important anticancer drugs.

266
329

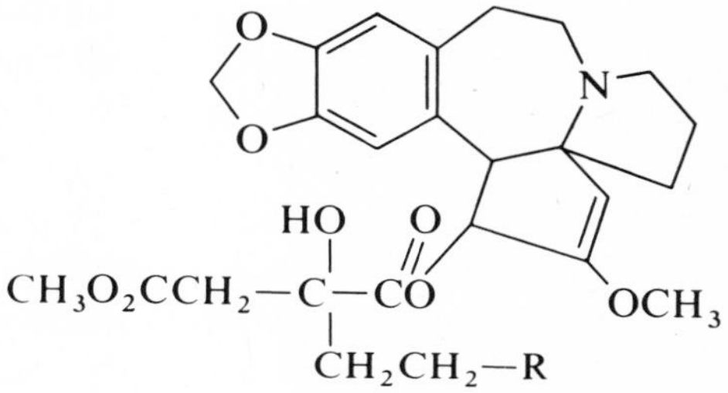

$$CH_3O_2CCH_2-\overset{\overset{\displaystyle HO}{|}}{\underset{\underset{\displaystyle CH_2CH_2-R}{|}}{C}}-\overset{\overset{\displaystyle O}{\|}}{C}O$$

$$\overset{\overset{\displaystyle OH}{|}}{}$$
106, R = —C(CH_3)_2
Harringtonine

LE T/C 137 (2 mg/kg)
PS T/C 294–405 (0.5–1 mg/kg)

107, R = —CH(CH_3)_2

Deoxyharringtonine

Similar LE and PS activity

$$\overset{\overset{\displaystyle OH}{|}}{}$$
108, R = —CH_2C(CH_3)_2
Homoharringtonine

LE T/C 142 (1 mg/kg)
PS T/C 244–338 (0.25–1 mg/kg)

Attention will now be directed to the quinoline- and isoquinoline-type biosynthetic products. By rigorous definition, some of these would not be considered alkaloids because of their optical inactivity. However, they are commonly termed alkaloids and are grouped here by virtue of their possible common intercalative properties. One of these important substances is ellipticine (**109**), and its 9-methoxy derivative was found mainly responsible for the antineoplastic response of extracts from the Apocynaceae species *Ochrosia moorei* F. Muell. and *Excavatia coccinea* (Trejs. and Bin.) Mgf. Both plants were uncovered as part of the NCI's collaborative program with the Australian CSIRO by Loder and Elmes.[75] Current requirements for ellipticine (**109**) are now being met by total synthesis.[75,192] From the original total synthesis reported by Woodward[435] in 1959, six separate total syntheses have been developed.

Acridine ring systems such as that exhibited by ellipticine are believed to owe part of their physiological activity to intercalative binding to DNA. Such an assumption has been considered for the planar ellipticine for about 10 years. Recently this hypothesis was subjected to a detailed study. Kohn and co-workers[194] found that effects of ellipticine on the sedimentation and viscosity of sheared DNA fragments suggest preferential binding to helical DNA by intercalation. A series of ellipticine analogues have been synthesized based on fit in a polynucleotide helix, and some of these have given T/C values in LE up to 292.[44] Similar synthetic manipulation with several of the more planar alkaloids to be reviewed shortly may also prove quite useful.

The simple acridine alkaloid (a group first discovered in the Rutaceae)[330] acronycine (**110**) has a surprisingly good range of antineoplastic activity and was found to inhibit growth in 12 of 17 different experimental tumor systems.[21,388] Acronycine was first isolated from bark of the Australian tree *Acronychia baueri* Schott. (Rutaceae) in 1948 by Hughes and colleagues.[165] The structure was determined in 1966 by Macdonald and Robertson[250] and biological, total synthetic,[21] and antineoplastic[388]

75

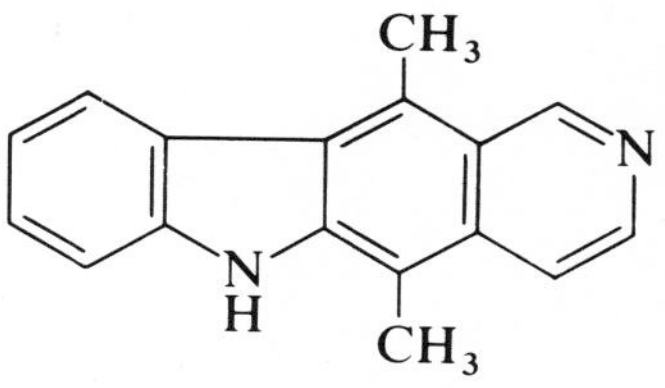

109

Ellipticine

LE T/C 172, PS T/C 204

250
388

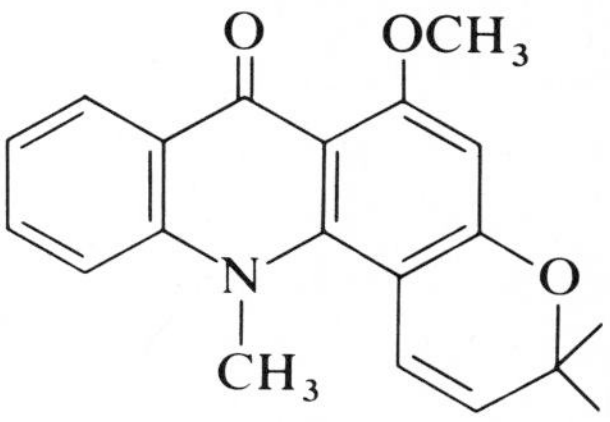

110

Acronycine

Active in 12 of 17 tumor systems

aspects have been pursued at the Lilly Research Laboratories.[389] Interestingly acronycine coprecipitated with polyvinylpyrrolidine displays a higher level of antineoplastic activity.

Emetine (**110a**) is an alkaloid that combines several structural features typical of the antineoplastic plant bases. Several Brazilian species of the family Rubiaceae, particularly *Cephaelis ipecacuanha* Rich. and *C. acuminata*, contain more than 2% alkaloids. The principal one is emetine (1.3%) accompanied by cephaeline (0.25%).[172] The use of ipecac root in native Indian medicine was recorded by a Brazilian priest in the 16th century. The root was more generally used in therapy beginning with the 17th century, particularly as an emetic and expectorant. In 1817, the isolation of emetine from ipecac root was described by Pelletier, and by 1912, the alkaloid was successfully employed in the treatment of amebic dysentery. Subsequently emetine became a valuable drug in the treatment of amebic hepatitis, which led us in 1965 to design emetine derivatives that might be of eventual use in the treatment of human hepatoma.[308] Meanwhile the NCI has had emetine under clinical development and initial results are now available.[270,372] A variety of total synthetic routes to emetine have been completed. Both emetine and camptothecin represent the most highly developed synthetic successes among the antineoplastic alkaloids.

The isoquinoline natural products nitidine chloride (**111**), fagaronine (**112**), and the coralyne salts (**113** and **114**) all bear a close resemblance, from the planar aromatic system to the quaternary ammonium salt. The most striking feature of these relatively simple biosynthetic products is their ability to inhibit markedly the progress of the PS leukemia. The relatively uncomplicated nature of these substances readily opens various avenues for synthetic modification, and it will be of interest to determine whether the parent compounds and any active derivatives are capable of intercalative binding to DNA.

The original isolation and structural determination of nitidine from the roots of *Zanthoxylum nitidum* were reported

270
308

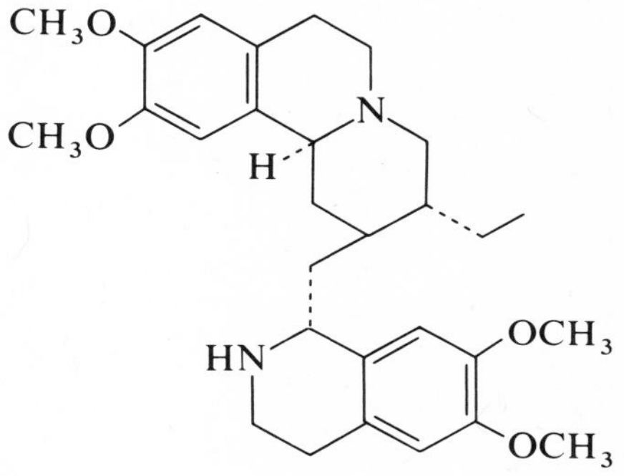

110a

Emetine

LE T/C 140, PS T/C 200

12
120

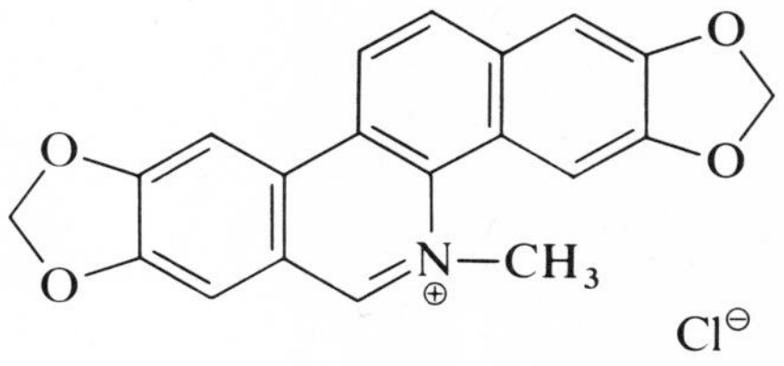

111

Nitidine chloride

LE T/C 134, PS T/C 197

264
399

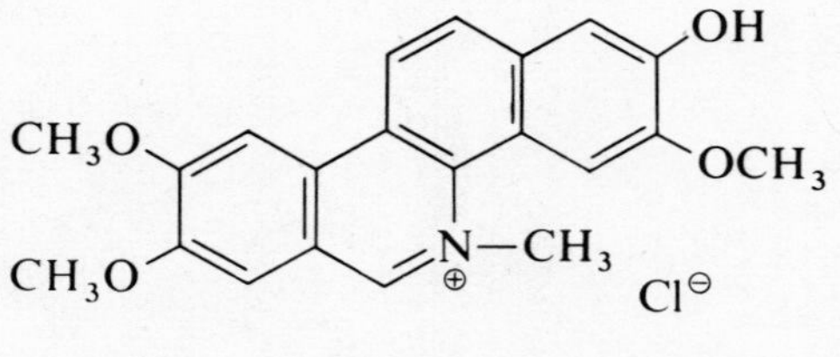

112
Fagaronine

PS T/C 265 (100 ml/kg)

439

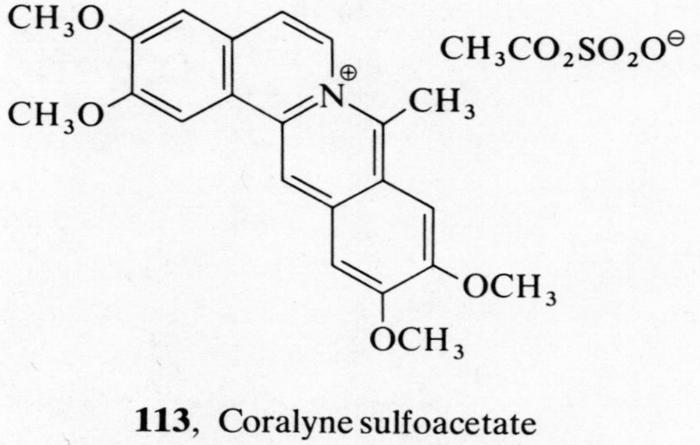

113, Coralyne sulfoacetate

LE T/C 140, PS T/C 190

114, Coralyne chloride

LE T/C 136, PS T/C 181

by the University of Hong Kong group of Arthur in 1958,[12] and a synthesis of dihydronitidine was completed the following year. The antineoplastic activity of nitidine chloride was reported by Wall in 1971.[415] The most recently discovered member, fagaronine, was isolated by the Farnsworth group[264,399] in 1972 from the Ghana plant *Fagara zanthoxyloides* Lam. (Rutaceae). A total synthesis of fagaronine was completed in 1974.[115]

The aporphines are truly alkaloids. One of these iso-quinoline derivatives (see also tetrandrine[400,185] in Volume 2), thalicarpine (**115**), was shown to be the cytotoxic constituent of *Thalictrum dasycarpum* Fisch. and Ave-Lall (Ranunculaceae) in 1963.[209] Later thalicarpine was found active against the WA carcinosarcoma, and in the life-span-extension method of evaluation, this substance gave a 285% increase at a dose of 64 mg/kg per day.[67] Thalicarpine apparently binds to DNA and inhibits its synthesis, as well as that of RNA and proteins. Total syntheses of thalicarpine have been completed[220,226] and this alkaloid has proceeded along in the NCI's programs to phase I clinical trial.[67] While thalicarpine has given evidence of human liver, kidney, cardiopulmonary, and CNS toxicity, the absence of myelosuppressive toxicity indicates that it might be of some use in combination with other anticancer drugs having that type of toxicity. No tumor responses were noted in the group of patients selected for phase I trial,[67] but further clinical study has been planned for both thalicarpine and tetrandrine.[139]

The amides and ansa macrolides are considered next. A recent review of macrolide antibiotics, particularly the erythromycin and carbomycin groups, has been prepared by Keller-Schierlein.[186] Plant amides with antineoplastic proper-ties range from the well-known and relatively simple colchicine (**116**)[206] to a glycoprotein of unknown structure obtained from an aqueous extract of *Mirabilis multiflora* (Nyctaginaceae) and active against S-180.[403] Another protein (cesalin) has been isolated from an aqueous extract of the Arizona plant *Caesal-pinia gilliesii* (Leguminosae).[404]

A brief history of colchicine and the secondary amine derivative demecolcine (**117**) has already been described in

70
145
226

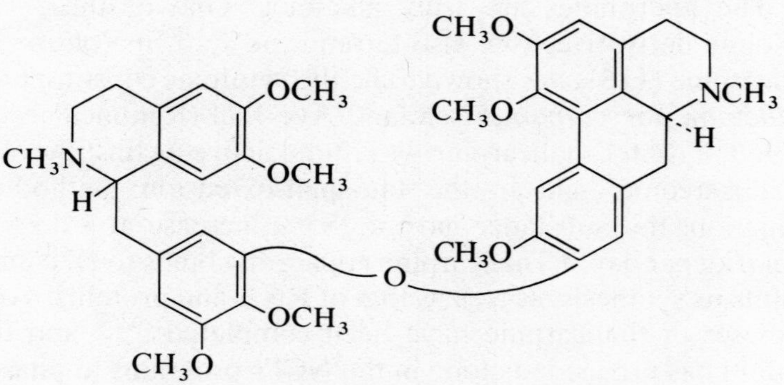

115

Thalicarpine

WA T/C 10, KB ED$_{50}$ 2.1 μg/ml

Chapter 2. A review of colchicine syntheses was prepared several years ago.[294] Hence discussion here will be limited to one of the most recent developments in this area. Kupchan and colleagues[206] have isolated colchicine, demecolcine, and 3-desmethylcolchicine (**118**) from the underground corms of the Dutch plant *Colchicum speciosum* Stev. (Liliaceae). Phenol **118** was found to exhibit activity against LE and cytotoxicity against the KB cell line. Such colchicine derivatives offer a new opportunity for structural modification. New investigations using contemporary methods might well capitalize on the long-standing lead provided by colchicine.

The maytansinoids represent an exciting new area of plant biosynthetic products for cancer chemotherapy. The Ethiopian plant *Maytenus ovatus* Loes. (Celastraceae), collected by Perdue and investigated by the Kupchan group,[224] has resulted in the isolation and structural determination of maytansine (**119**), an ansa macrolide with a broad spectrum of *in vivo* anticancer activity. At the time of writing, maytansine was in phase I clinical trial by the NCI.

Meanwhile the Wall group[422] has isolated and characterized colubrinol (**121**), a closely related antineoplastic ansa macrolide from the Rhamnaceae plant *Colubrina texensis* Gray. The most promising antineoplastic activity of these ansa macrolides has inspired a further study leading to maytanvaline (**120**) from *Maytenus buchananii* (Loes) R. Wilczek.[223] The newest advance has entailed isolation and structural determination of the highly active maytanacine (**122**) from *Putterlickia verrucosa* Szyszyl. (Celastraceae).[205] Structure/activity studies available at present point to the possibility that minor variations in the ester group at C-3 will not markedly change the PS activity. On the other hand, the maytansid obtained by the removal of the ester and the elimination of the oxygen group results in a pronounced reduction in PS activity. Attempts at the total synthesis of maytansine are already in progress.[265]

Maytansine is very effective by the intraperitoneal route with mice carrying the vincristine-sensitive P-388 leukemia in ascites form but has proved ineffective against the vincristine-

206

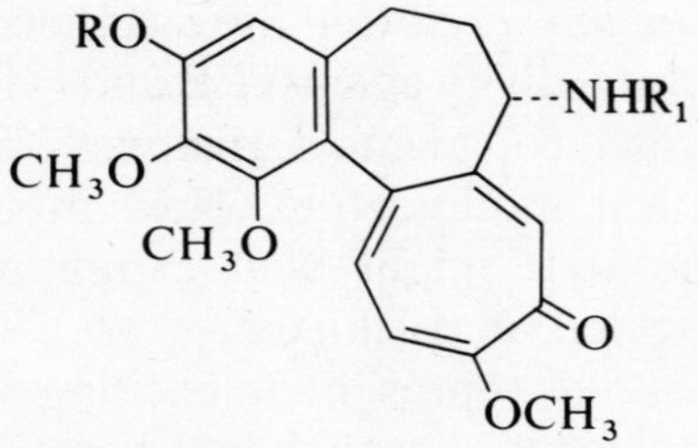

116, R = —CH$_3$, R$_1$ = COCH$_3$

Colchicine

PS active

117, R = —CH$_3$, R$_1$ = —CH$_3$

Demecolcine

LE T/C 139, PS T/C 150

118, R = H, R$_1$ = COCH$_3$

3-Desmethylcolchicine

LE active

205
223
224
422

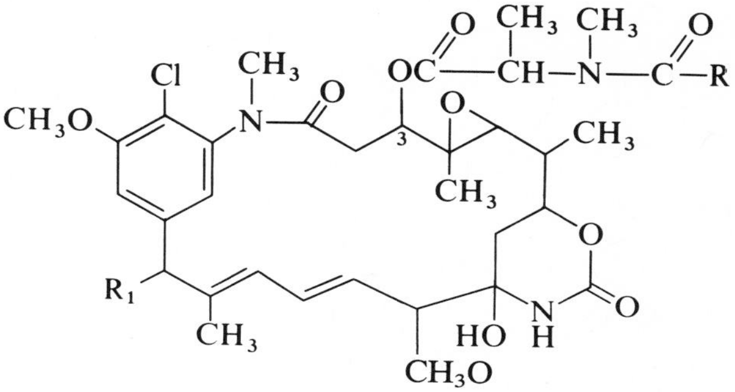

119, R = —CH₃, R₁ = H

Maytansine

PS T/C 200, B1 T/C 151, LL T/C 130

KB ED₅₀ 1 × 10⁻⁵ μg/ml

120, R = —CH₂CH(CH₃)₂, R₁ = H

Maytanvaline

PS active

121, R = —CH(CH₃)₂, R₁ = —OH

Colubrinol

PS active, KB ED₅₀ 1 × 10⁻⁴ μg/ml

122, C-3, OCOCH₃, R₁ = H

Maytanacine

PS T/C 230 (100 μg/kg)

205
223
224
422

119, $R = -CH_3$, $R_1 = H$

Maytansine

PS T/C 200, B1 T/C 151, LL T/C 130

KB ED$_{50}$ 1×10^{-5} μg/ml

120, $R = -CH_2CH(CH_3)_2$, $R_1 = H$

Maytanvaline

PS active

121, $R = -CH(CH_3)_2$, $R_1 = -OH$

Colubrinol

PS active, KB ED$_{50}$ 1×10^{-4} μg/ml

122, C-3, $OCOCH_3$, $R_1 = H$

Maytanacine

PS T/C 230 (100 μg/kg)

resistant line.[432] So far, maytansine seems to exert its activity by inhibition of DNA synthesis.[432] The ansa macrolides should have a bright future in cancer chemotherapy, and hopefully maytansine or a related substance will become of great clinical utility. At the very least, the substances will prove valuable as biochemical probes[340] and starting points for synthetic manipulations.

Fungi and Other Lower Plant Biosynthetic Products

The ubiquitous lower plants commonly known as mildews, molds, mushrooms, puffballs, rusts, and smuts are members of the fungi group and represent exceedingly large numbers of different species. By definition, the fungi lack chlorophyll and have a threadlike plant body or mycelium. Consequently the fungi are dependent upon other living organisms for food, and some, such as the mushrooms and puffballs, form a compact mycelium of substantial size. Three great classes of fungi are recognized, namely, the Ascomycetes, the Basidiomycetes, and the Phycomycetes. The *Fungi imperfecti* do not represent a homogeneous class but rather a large number of species that have lost their ability of sexual reproduction.

The morels and truffles represent the larger edible forms of Ascomycetes (septate mycelium, asexual reproduction). Many mildews and molds comprise smaller forms, such as the genera *Penicillium* and *Aspergillus*. The Basidiomycetes (septate mycelium, complicated reproduction from asexual to sexual) contain the bracket fungi, mushrooms, puffballs, rusts, smuts, and other types. The Phycomycetes (nonseptate mycelium, asexual reproduction) include the plant parasite *Phytophthora infestans* (potato blight), the common bread mold *Rhizopus nigricans*, and the water mold *Saprolegnia*, parasitic of fish.

One class (Schizomycetes) in the lowest division of the plant kingdom contains the bacteria. The Schizomycetes class is divided into five orders of unicellular plants. The order Actinomycetales are funguslike bacteria, and the family Actinomycetaceae contains the genus *Actinomyces*, whose members more closely resemble the *Fungi imperfecti* than bacteria. Both the *Actinomyces* and the members of the genus *Streptomyces* of the related family Streptomycetaceae have been extensively explored for antibiotic and antineoplastic constituents. The astronomical number of other lower plants that have never been evaluated for antineoplastic components staggers the imagination and offers a great number of exciting prospects for the future.

The microorganism and antineoplastic agents selected for discussion in this chapter are those with substantial *in vivo* activity and are either already in clinical use or being considered for clinical trial. Other microorganism components with cytotoxic and/or lesser antineoplastic properties are included in the tabular survey of Volume 2. So far, the anticancer antibiotics seem to be organizable into a relatively small number of structural types. The classifications devised for this chapter have been utilized to emphasize structure/activity correlations. The result is a series of terpene epoxides (and macrolides), aflatoxin-like dihydrofurans, quinones, alkylating units (aziridine, β-chloroethylamine), modified (heterocyclic ring) nucleosides, anthracyclines and abbreviated anthracycline types, *N*-nitroso amides and amines, modified amino acids and diazoketones, chromopeptides, peptides with unusual amino acids, and finally low to high molecular weight proteins.

As would be expected from such distinct structural differences, the anticancer antibiotics inhibit cell growth by a variety of mechanisms. The better-known representatives from each classification have been found to interfere with DNA, RNA, or protein syntheses and/or the normal function of cell membranes and mitochondria. With the more useful antibiotics, the action is very specific. For example, penicillin interferes with synthesis of the bacterial cell wall. Others are much less specific and some of the antineoplastic antibiotics interfere with both normal and abnormal cell growth. Fortunately the better antitumor antibiotics yield a cumulative effect more detrimental to neoplastic cells.

The terpenoid mycophenolic acid (**123**) was probably the first antibiotic to be isolated from a fungus. In 1896, Gosio isolated a substance from *Penicillium glaucum* that suppressed the growth of the anthrax bacillus.[30] A compound believed to be the same was isolated from *Penicillium stoloniferum* in 1913 and given the present name mycophenolic acid. By 1948, the structure was known,[30,31] and a total synthesis was reported by Birch in 1969, followed by another in 1972.[48] Eventually the antineoplastic behavior of mycophenolic acid became known and a clinical trial was begun in England.[176] When one is looking at the history of mycophenolic acid, it is interesting to consider that 44 years elapsed between the original discovery of antibiotic activity and the first application of a *Penicillium* antibiotic (e.g., **124**) in medicine. The tragically slow recognition of practical medical applications for the initial observations in 1896 is certainly disconcerting. The possible application of this historically significant metabolite or a derivative in cancer chemotherapy continues to be of interest.

The diepoxy mold metabolite fumagillin (**125**) was isolated from *Aspergillus fumigatus* in 1951 and later found to be a potentially useful amebicide and antineoplastic agent.[393] The structure was reported by Tarbell and colleagues[393] 10 years later, and some 10 years thereafter, a total synthesis of the racemic metabolite was completed by Corey and Snider.[66] Another type of terpenoid epoxide mold metabolite is illustrated by verrucarin A (**126**).

The soil fungi *Myrothecium verrucaria* and *M. roridum* in the Moniliales order of the *Fungi imperfecti* are parasitic on tomato leaves, violets, and other common plants and produce a very active cellulase. In an extensive study by Tamm and co-workers at the University of Basel, the antifungal and cytotoxic constituents of these molds were found to be verrucarin A (**126**) and a series of related substances.[392] The

176

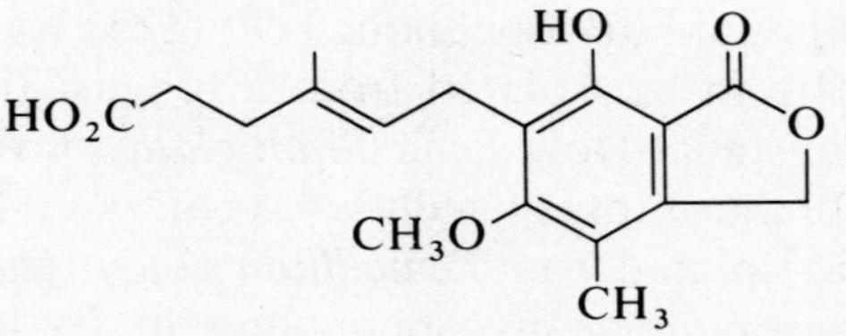

123

Mycophenolic acid

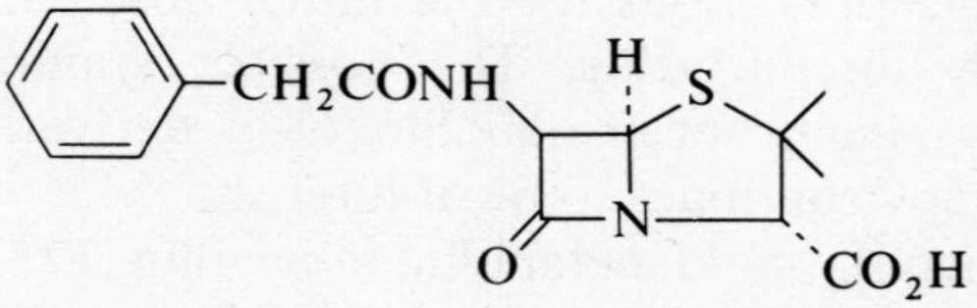

124

Penicillin G

66
145
393

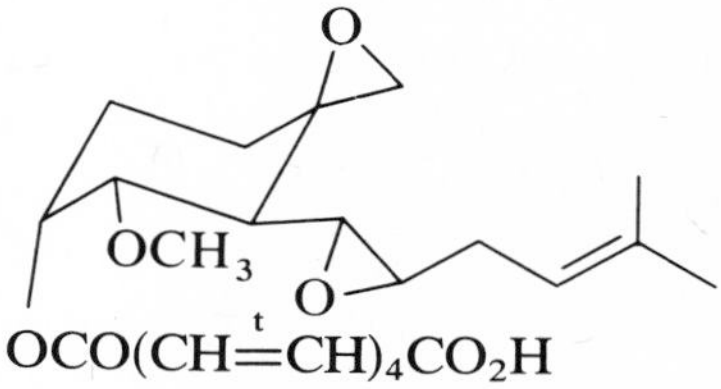

125

Fumagillin

SA T/C 20 (12 mg/kg)
EA and CA active

133
392

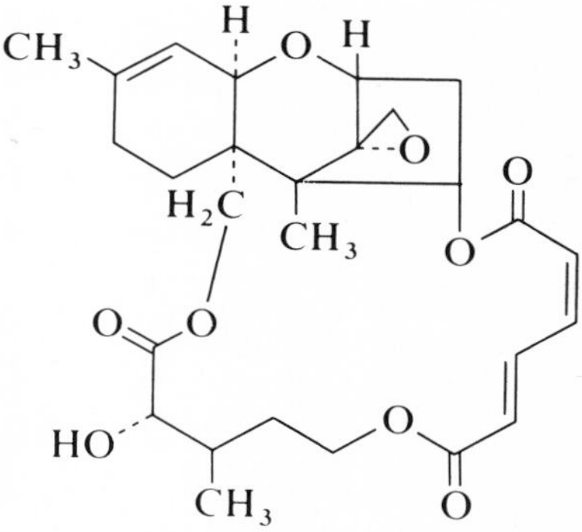

126

Verrucarin A

WA and S-37 active

macrocyclic lactone **126** was found to have antifungal activity, to show slight inhibition against gram-negative bacteria, to show antiviral activity against *Herpes simplex* virus strain (HSV), and even to have insecticidal action against the Mexican bean beetle. Of most interest here was the antiviral activity, the cytotoxicity (ED_{50} 6×10^{-4}) against the murine P-815 cell line, and the *in vivo* antitumor activity. Catalytic reduction of the olefin system (**126**) causes a substantial loss of activity, while reduction of the epoxide leads to a complete loss of activity.[392] In 1965, a group at Sandoz[248] disclosed isolation of the diacetate ester of the parent alcohol verrucarol and designated it anguidin (**127**). The latter substance was obtained from *Fusarium* species and is now of interest as a possible candidate for cancer chemotherapy clinical trial.

The molds, common to various human food materials, have probably been responsible for toxic and/or lethal effects from at least the beginnings of food gathering and storage. Such mycotoxicosis was already known in approximately 760 B.C. and is mentioned in the Book of Amos. Until about 1960, the best-known example was that of ergotism resulting from the ingestion of bread containing rye bearing the fungus *Claviceps purpurea*. In 1960, the death of some 100,000 turkeys on farms in England led to recognition of the so-called turkey X disease as a mycotoxicosis caused by peanut meal infected with the mold *Aspergillus flavus* Link and Fries. Subsequently this mold was found to produce a number of very toxic metabolites now known as the aflatoxins (*a* for genus, *fla* for species, and *toxins*). The major metabolite was found to be an exceedingly potent carcinogen designated aflatoxin B_1 (**1**), which has proved to be the most potent liver carcinogen so far uncovered. About 10 years ago, aflatoxin B_1 and companion substances were found to be responsible for the liver cancer of hatchery rainbow trout. Seven other very toxic aflatoxins closely related to aflatoxin B_1 (**1**) have been isolated and characterized.[345] More recently, the major metabolite of B_1 was isolated, designated aflatoxin Q_1, and synthesized.[42]

In 1954, a Japanese group isolated sterigmatocystin[276] and the structure was determined in 1962.[148,149,345] By 1966, the carcinogenicity of sterigmatocystin was known,[162] but fortunately it is much less than that of the aflatoxins. The University of Liverpool group, ably led by Holker,[161] isolated and characterized 5-methoxysterigmatocystin (**128**) from a mutant strain of *Aspergillus versicolor*. The 5-methoxy derivative **128** has proved very effective against a series of key rodent tumor systems in the NCI's programs and is of interest for possible clinical application. However, in this series of fungal metabolites, the carcinogenic possibilities have to be carefully assessed.

Mitomycin C (**129**) and sangivamycin (**130**) are representative of the quinone and nucleoside classes[76] of anticancer antibiotics that have been under investigation for about 15 years. The original isolation of mitomycin C from *Streptomyces caesipitosus* by a Japanese group in 1958 was quickly followed by a series of structural determinations concluded by Stevens and colleagues.[381] Clinical trials of mitomycin C have been continuing, and in 1974, it was approved by the U.S. Food and Drug Administration for normal use in medical practice (see Table 1). Sangivamycin (**130**) was isolated from a *Streptomyces* sp. and structurally identified by Rao in the NCI's program formerly at Pfizer.[335] Pactamycin[28] (from *Streptomyces pactum* var. *Pactum*) and sparsomycin[36,326] (from *Streptomyces sparsogenes* var. *Sparsogenes*) represent two partially identified antitumor antibiotics isolated as part of the NCI's program at the Upjohn Company.

Discovery of the mitomycins nicely demonstrated that biosynthetic processes in nature can yield very reactive substituents, such as the aziridine group (alkylating properties) of mitomycin C. More recently, a biosynthetic analogy for the well-known bis(2-chloroethyl)amine alkylating agents— namely, a constituent of *Streptomyces griseoluteus* was designated 593A by a Merck Sharp and Dohme group.[11] After the present review was in press, we established by X-ray crystallographic methods structure **131** for 593A.[324a] This

248

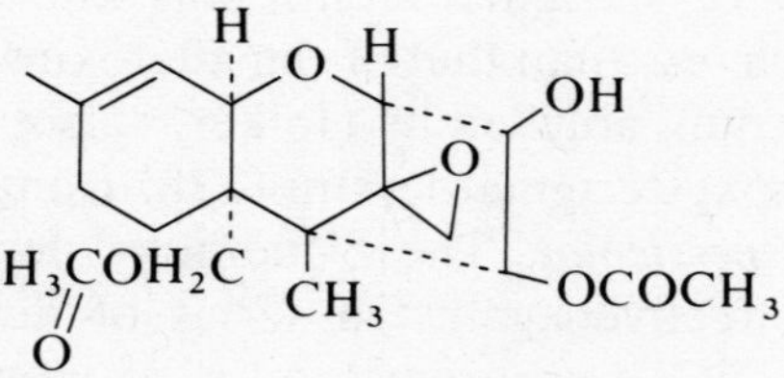

127

Anguidin

LE T/C 144, PS T/C 207

148
149
161
434

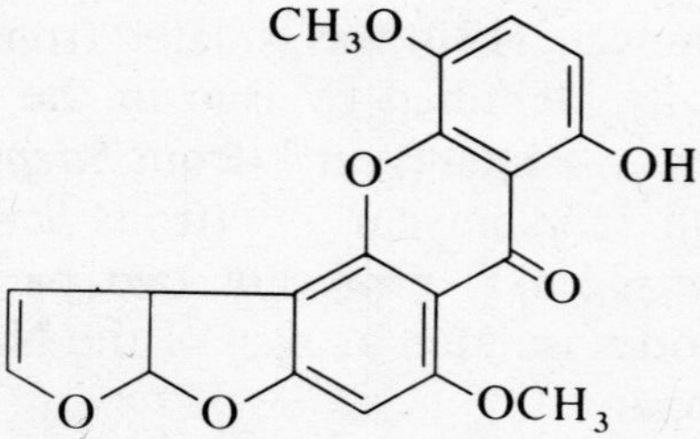

128

5-Methoxysterigmatocystin

LE T/C 160, PS T/C 245
B1 T/C 134, LL T/C 139

118
381
425

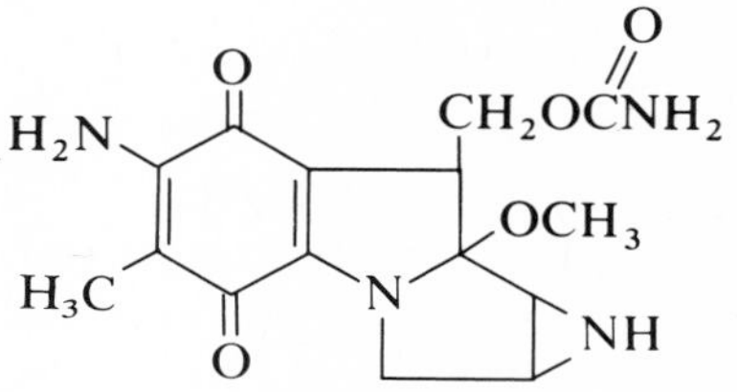

129

Mitomycin C

LE T/C 200, PS T/C 250, B1 T/C 142 (1 mg/kg)

Porfiromycin (*N*-methyl mitomycin C)

335

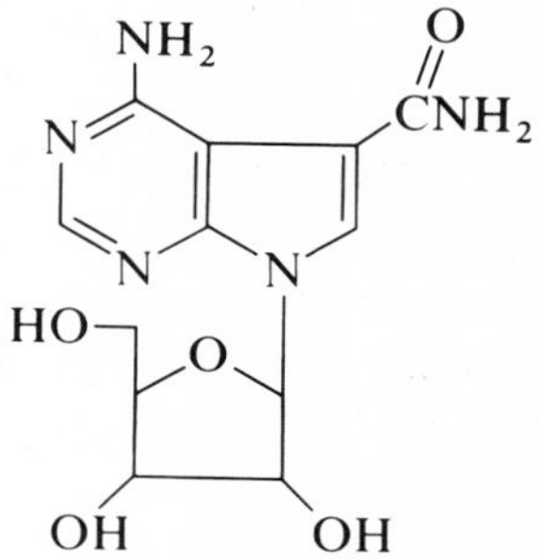

130

Sangivamycin

LE T/C 167, PS T/C 190

piperazinedione is currently under clinical investigation, and efforts to develop a convenient total synthesis are under way in our laboratory. Because 593A (**131**) is also a derivative of glycine, it should also be considered among the amino acid derivatives discussed below.

The well-known tetracycline antibiotics, such as oxytetracycline isolated from *Streptomyces rimosus*, caused a further intensification of studies with *Streptomyces*. Undoubtedly this emphasis upon *Streptomyces* played a crucial role in speeding the development of the anthracycline antitumor antibiotics. At the same time, the pioneering chemical investigations of Brockmann, Woodward, and Muxfeldt greatly assisted in advancement of this field.[38] The antineoplastic antibiotics of this class extend from the tricyclic but complex mithramycin (**132**) and chromomycin A$_3$ (**133**) to the tetracyclic but relatively simple anthracycline glycosides of the adriamycin (**136**) type.

The substance named aureolic acid (**132**), originally isolated in 1953, was rediscovered by Rao in a *Streptomyces* species and named mithramycin.[337] Similarly the antibiotic called LA-7017, uncovered in 1958, was also found to be identical with aureolic acid.[16] Thus aureolic acid is the formally correct name, but since this compound is better known as mithramycin, this name will be used here. Since the original discovery of aureolic acid, about 20 related antibiotics have been isolated from *Streptomyces* and *Actinomyces* species.[373]

The structure of mithramycin was determined by the Kolosov group[16] in Moscow. A confirmational analysis of their structural proposal by this reviewer suggests that structure **132** is a convenient representation of mithramycin. Inspection of the glycoside components of mithramycin indicates that the D-olivose portion must be identical with the corresponding chromose portion of chromomycin A$_3$ (**133**). The latter cancer chemotherapeutic drug was isolated from *Streptomyces griseus* by Shibata and co-workers in 1960, and the structure was reported in 1967.[268] Chromomycin A$_3$ has been in clinical use in Japan for some time in combination with other antineoplastic agents.[405] Mithramycin has been in clinical trial at various times

11

131

593A

LE T/C > 200
RO active

16
117
118
337

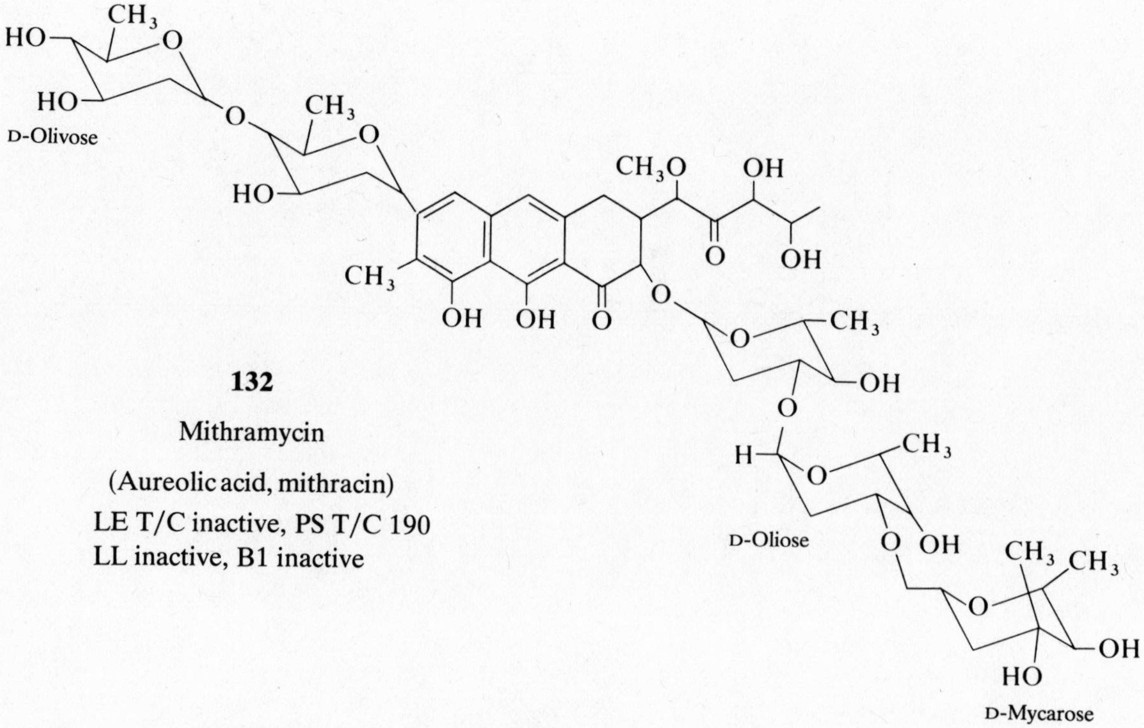

132

Mithramycin

(Aureolic acid, mithracin)

LE T/C inactive, PS T/C 190

LL inactive, B1 inactive

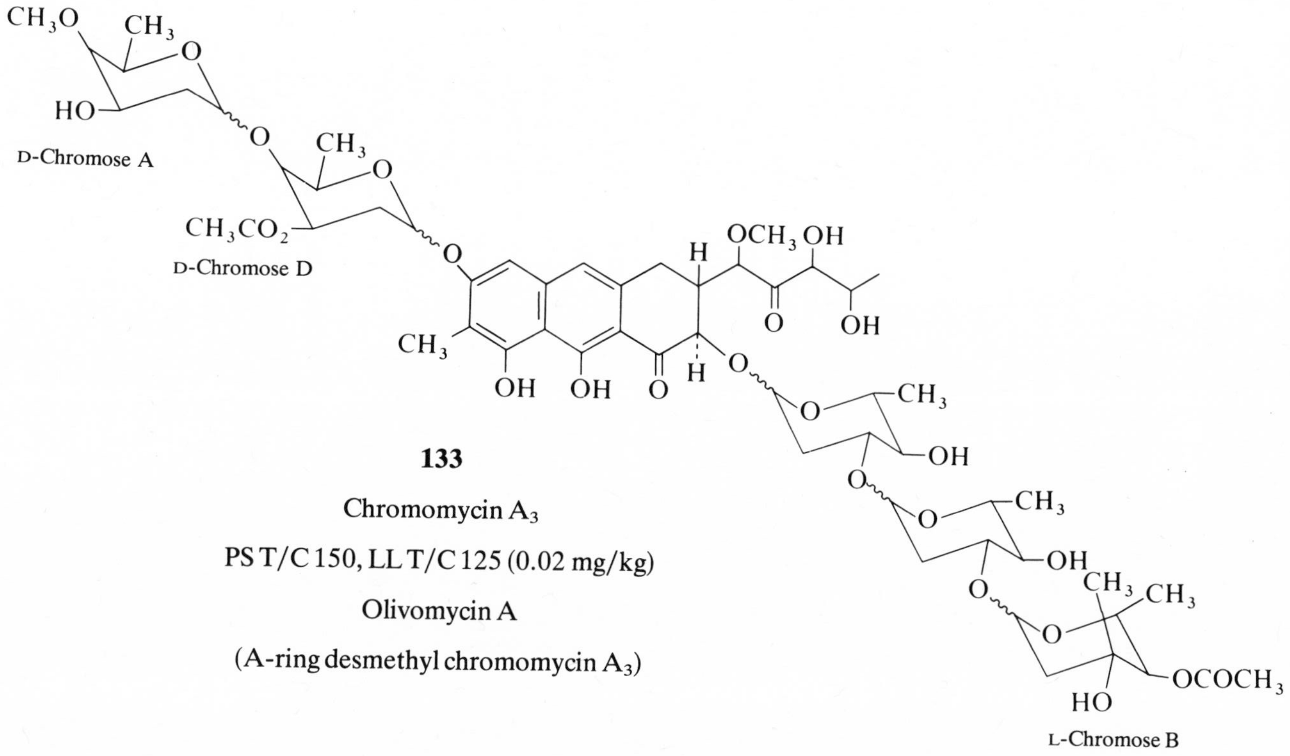

268

133

Chromomycin A$_3$

PST/C150, LL T/C125 (0.02 mg/kg)

Olivomycin A

(A-ring desmethyl chromomycin A$_3$)

in the United States from the late 1960's. Unfortunately, as noted below, neither compound has yet demonstrated outstanding clinical utility.

Mithramycin seems to inhibit synthesis of DNA as well as DNA-directed synthesis of RNA. There is some indication that mithramycin may stabilize the secondary structure of DNA through bridge formation linking complementary strands of the DNA helix. Clinically mithramycin is a very toxic drug, and fatalities of up to 10% attributable to mithramycin have been experienced in some clinical studies.[246] In these cases, death was caused by hemorrhage, but this most serious limitation can be minimized by the reduction of the dose to about 50 μg/kg per dose on an every-other-day schedule. By this means, the useful cancer chemotherapeutic effects upon testical embryonal carcinoma have been preserved. So far, mithramycin seems most useful for testicular cancer of the embryonal type and for the treatment of hypercalcelia and hypercalciuria resulting from neoplastic disease. Mithramycin has been available for use in such practice since 1970.

A phase I clinical study of chromomycin A_3 was begun by the Moertel group[197] several years ago, and the dose-limiting toxicity was found to be acute renal tubular damage, which produced azotemia and protein urea. More recently, the same group studied the application of chromomycin A_3 in advanced colorectal carcinoma. In the 27 patients evaluated, no evidence of therapeutic utility was observed.[269] Perhaps other dosage schedules will be more productive, and/or other types of human neoplastic diseases may be more sensitive to this cancer chemotherapeutic agent. Alternatively present clinical results may be a true reflection of the rather marginal activity shown by chromomycin A_3 in several of the NCI's key experimental tumor systems. Hopefully clinical evaluation of the closely related olivomycin A (the ring A desmethyl derivative of chromomycin A_3) will be more productive.[373]

In the tetracyclic series, granaticin A (**134**) is one of the newest entries. Although this antitumor antibiotic was isolated by the Swiss group of Prelog in 1957 from *Streptomyces olivaceus*, its activity against murine leukemia was not known

57

134

Granaticin A

PS T/C 166 (1.5 mg/kg)

until 1975.[57] A possibly related quinone antitumor (Ehrlich carcinoma in mice) antibiotic of unknown structure ($C_{19}H_{14}O_6$) was recently isolated from a *Chainia* species of Actinomycetes obtained from a marine mud collected in the Japanese Sagami Bay.[289] While we made a small collection of marine muds in 1971 to evaluate the possibility of locating microorganisms producing anticancer agents, the study reported by Okazaki[289] probably represents the first isolation of such compounds from marine microorganisms. As with most other branches of lower plant life, such marine microorganisms offer intriguing possibilities for the future.

In 1957, a Farmitalia group cultured a soil microorganism from southern Italy and isolated a red pigment-producing colony. The microorganism was later named *Streptomyces peucetius* and found to produce daunomycin (**135**).[113] Attempts at inducing mutation in *S. peucetius* and isolating variant strains led to the formation of an aerial mycelium with blue-green to gray-green coloration. The new organism was designated *S. peucetius* var. *caesius*, and it was found to produce the 14-hydroxy derivative of daunomycin now known as adriamycin (**136**).[113] Clinical trials of both daunomycin and adriamycin began in the late 1960's, and the structures were elucidated by Arcamone and co-workers.[6,9] Meanwhile syntheses of the aglycone daunomycinone and the carbohydrate unit daunosamine have been completed. Both components have been combined to yield daunomycin, and further chemical conversion to adriamycin has completed the overall structural assignments for these anthracyclines.[1,8,189,254,433]

Dose-limiting cardiotoxicity (congestive heart failure) has severely restricted the clinical application of daunomycin.[305,125] The upper limit of safety with this toxicity for adriamycin is a cumulative dose of 500 mg/m^2 in children and up to 720 mg/m^2 in adults. However, in a recent study, two out of four patients who had cumulative doses of 600 mg/m^2 of adriamycin experienced congestive heart failure.[23] In general, adriamycin treatment can also be limited by hematologic toxicity and alopecia. Nausea and stomatitis are also encountered but are generally predictable and reversible. Clinical application of adriamycin in neoplastic disease has been especially encouraging, and objective responses are well established in adenocarcinoma of the breast, Wilms' tumor, bronchogenic carcinoma, neuroblastoma, malignant sarcomas, and hematologic malignancies.[121,122,347] By way of illustration, 36 patients with disseminated sarcomas were recently treated with adriamycin at a dose of 60 mg/m^2 over a 3-week period. Of these patients, 9% went into complete remission and 32% into partial remission, and improvement was noted in 21% for medium durations of 37, 18, and 15 weeks. In each of the responding patients, overall survival was prolonged.[23] Clinical interest in adriamycin has been so intense that a recent complete issue of *Cancer Chemotherapy Reports* was devoted to this cancer chemotherapeutic drug.[46] Generally speaking, daunomycin is one of the most effective single agents for induction of remission in acute lymphoblastic and myeloblastic leukemia, while adriamycin is more effective against human solid tumors.

Both daunomycin and adriamycin are known to bind with nucleic acids and disrupt DNA and RNA syntheses. Apparently the planar anthracycline nucleus fits well by intercalation into the DNA double helix (thereby distorting the polymer) with consequent interference in biochemical utilization of the distorted DNA. Presumably adriamycin functions by an analogous mechanism and also inhibits nucleic acid synthesis. However, the surprising difference in *in vivo* antineoplastic activity has recently been attributed to an observation that daunomycin may more readily pass through cell membranes.[15] Substantial attempts have been under way in recent years, particularly in the NCI's programs, to develop structural modifications of adriamycin even more effective against human solid neoplasms. Eventually structural modification should lead to substances with less hazardous cardiotoxicity and greater antineoplastic activity.

In 1973, a promising anthracycline cancer chemotherapeutic agent designated carminomycin 1 (**137**) was reported by Gause and co-workers.[109] The new antibiotic was isolated from

305
355

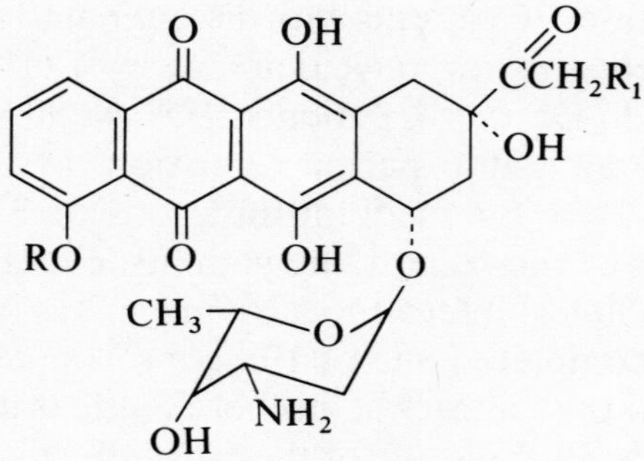

135, R = —CH$_3$, R$_1$ = H

Daunomycin
(Daunorubicin)

LE T/C 158, PS T/C 227, B1 T/C 260

136, R = —CH$_3$, R$_1$ = OH

Adriamycin

LE T/C 164, PS > 300, B1 T/C 300

137, R = R$_1$ = H

Carminomycin 1

LE some cures

Actinomadura carminata sp. nov. and more recently from *A. cremeospinus* sp. nov.[107] and assigned a desmethyl daunomycin structure.[35] Carminomycin 1 (**137**) has been found more effective than either daunomycin or adriamycin in inhibiting DNA synthesis[154] and in inhibiting growth of the LE leukemia.[35] In other preliminary animal studies, carminomycin 1 was found to suppress (95%) the growth of a murine bronchogenic lung carcinoma,[35] to give evidence of less severe cardiotoxicity (rabbit evaluation), and to be better absorbed from the gastrointestinal tract than daunomycin.[108] By means of an X-ray crystallographic study, we have assigned structure **137** to carminomycin 1.[305] Meanwhile our group found that an antitumor antibiotic arising from the former NCI program at Bristol and continued by the Wall group[424] is, in fact, carminomycin 1.[305] In this case, the specimen of carminomycin 1 was obtained from a *Streptomyces*. Carminomycin 1 is now undergoing clinical trial in the Soviet Union. Given the clinical differences experienced already between such closely related substances as daunomycin and adriamycin, it would seem that carminomycin 1 will have different and hopefully better clinical activity. Unfortunately daunomycin has a rather narrow therapeutic index; hopefully carminomycin 1 will not have this limitation.

Streptozotocin (**138**) is representative of a completely different class of antitumor antibiotic. Here, the *N*-nitroso group with an appropriate hydrophilic carrier seems primarily responsible for the antineoplastic effects. Streptozotocin was originally obtained by an Upjohn group in the late 1950's from *Streptomyces achromogenes* var. 128.[158] *In vitro* screening indicated that the compound was active against both gram-negative and gram-positive bacteria. Later *N*-nitrosourea **138** was found to inhibit progression of the LE leukemia and interfere with DNA synthesis in cells derived from both bacteria and mammals. A recent study of streptozotocin labeled with ^{14}C and ^{3}H and given to patients with advanced cancer indicated that it remained in the plasma over the first 3 hours. Radioactive metabolic products were present for longer than 24 hours.[2]

Some 15% of the streptozotocin administered was detected in the urine along with three major metabolites.

Streptozotocin is not myelosuppressive at dose levels useful against human neoplastic disease. Accordingly this *N*-nitrosourea has been of interest for use in patients with bone marrow suppression resulting from prior chemotherapy and/or radiation treatment.[287] When animal toxicity studies pointed to the diabetogenic effects of streptozotocin, it was subsequently evaluated as a chemotherapeutic drug for human metastatic insulinoma (better known as a metastatic islet-cell tumor of the pancreas) and was found active against this particular neoplastic disease. Recently its use against acute lymphocytic leukemia has been abandoned at the Baltimore Cancer Research Center of the NCI.[287] However, the substance may have some eventual utility in malignant lymphoma.[287]

From a chemical standpoint, streptozotocin is simply a glucose derivative of the well-known organic chemical reagent *N*-methylnitrosourea. The latter substance was early detected as an active agent in the NCI's exploratory screening of synthetic compounds. More recently, *N*-methylnitrosourea has received an initial clinical trial in the Soviet Union. This writer saw one patient with malignant melanoma in the Institute of Clinical and Experimental Oncology in Moscow who had been very successfully treated with this very reactive substance. Synthetic modification of streptozotocin and synthesis of related substances has been under way for some time.[251] A recent series of streptozotocin analogues prepared by Acton and colleagues in the NCI's program at Stanford Research Institute has led to LE T/C values up to 220.[105]

The microbiologically produced amino acids with antineoplastic activity have for the most part proved to be *N*-nitroso, oxime, and diazoketone derivatives. An interesting example is that of L(−)-alanosine (**139**) obtained by a Lepetit group from *Streptomyces alanosinicus* in 1964.[241,397] A synthesis of racemic alanosine has been completed.[90] Currently this alanine derivative is supplied by Dow-Lepetit and is of interest to the NCI. The diazoketone type of amino acid derivative was

118
158
434

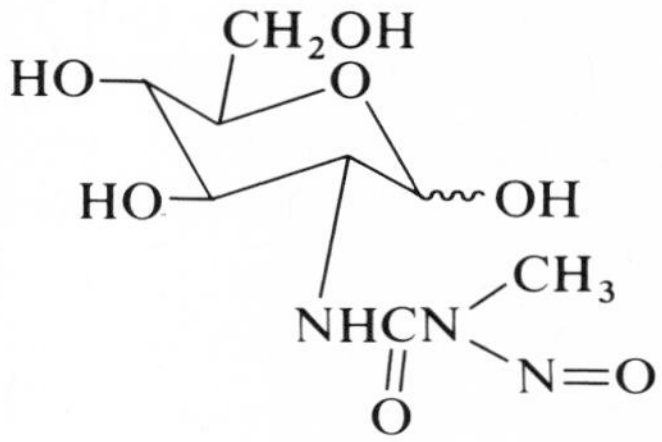

138

Streptozotocin

LE T/C 160, PS T/C 154
LL T/C 121 (200 mg/kg)

38

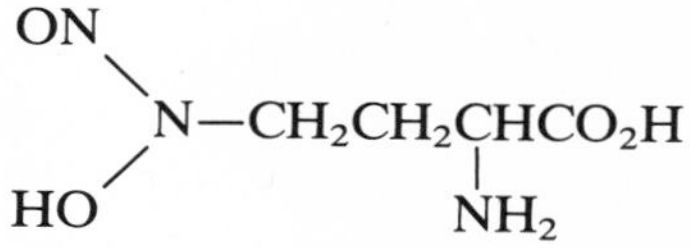

139

L(−)-Alanosine

LE T/C 182, PS T/C 181

first reported in 1954 by the Sloan-Kettering investigators who isolated azaserine (**140**). Unfortunately azaserine has not proved to be very useful in the clinic.[277] A related biosynthetic product, 6-diazo-5-oxo-L-norleucine (DON), has also not proved to be a practical drug.[89] However, azotomycin (**141**) can be tolerated in humans at five times the maximum dosage of DON, and it is interesting to note that while the maximum tolerated dose in mice and dogs of diazoketone **141** is 0.1 mg/kg per day for 14 days, most humans can tolerate 2 mg/kg per day for 7–14 days.[428] Of particular importance is the fact that azotomycin has shown activity against human gastrointestinal carcinoma and various soft-tissue sarcomas. The original isolation of azotomycin from *Streptomyces ambofaciens* was reported by Rao at Pfizer in 1961.[336] Other glutamic acid and glutaric acid derivatives, such as the glutarimide antibiotics (e.g., streptovitacin A), have been isolated and found effective against various experimental tumor systems.[277,405] Some of these substances are included in the tabular survey of Volume 2.

Two representatives of a new *Streptomyces*-derived amino acid with antineoplastic activity have been uncovered in the NCI's program at Upjohn.[256,257] Both were isolated from *S. sviceus* and found to have the usual 3-chloro-isoxazole system shown by structures **142** and **143**. The 4-hydroxy derivative **143** is a minor constituent of the metabolic products. Structures **142** and **143** were established by X-ray crystallographic methods, and biological studies are in progress.[129,258]

Actinomycin D (**144**) was the first peptide antineoplastic agent to receive extensive study. A brief view of the history was given in Chapter 2. The chemistry of actinomycins was reviewed in 1974.[47,273] The use of actinomycin D as a curative treatment for Wilms' tumor and gestational choriocarcinoma (70–90% cure rate) is now well established.[47] A recent study by Goldin and Johnson[118] of actinomycin D against experimental tumor systems was focused on establishing models for predicting future applications in combination chemotherapy. Chromopeptide **144** was found to be highly active against the PS, B1, adenocarcinoma 755, and Ridgway osteogenic sarcoma. In the

118
382

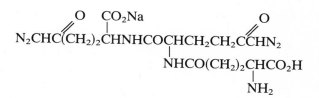

140

Azaserine

LE T/C 142 (54 mg/kg)

428

$$N_2CHC(CH_2)_2CHNHCOCHCH_2CH_2CCHN_2$$

141

Azotomycin

LE T/C 168, PS T/C 220
WA and SA very active

256

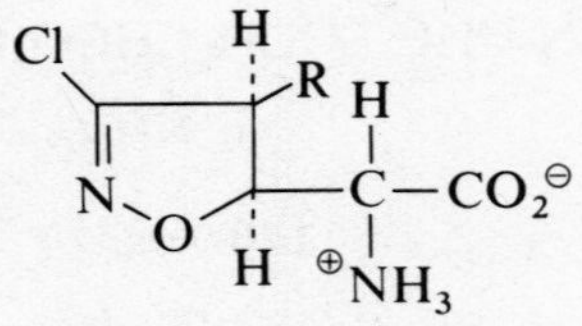

142, R = H (NSC 163, 501)

LE T/C 150 (1.5 mg/kg)

143, R = OH (NSC 176, 324)

LE T/C 150 (1.5 mg/kg)
and 161 (50 mg/kg)

47
118
262

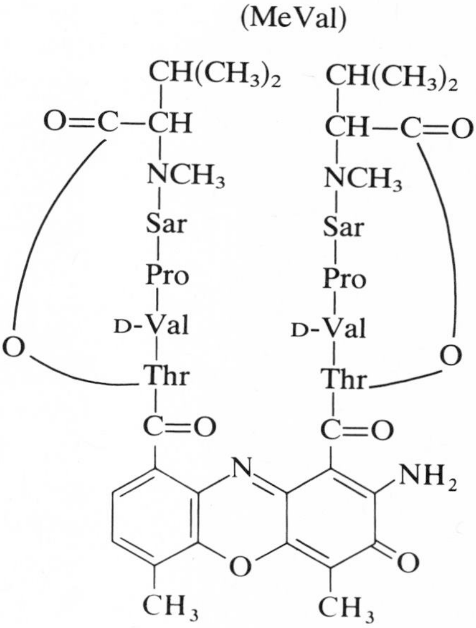

(MeVal)

$$\text{CH(CH}_3)_2 \qquad \text{CH(CH}_3)_2$$

$$\text{O=C—CH} \qquad \text{CH—C=O}$$

|
NCH₃   NCH₃
|
Sar   Sar
|
Pro   Pro
|
D-Val   D-Val
|
O   Thr   Thr   O
|
C=O   C=O

N

NH₂

O

O

CH₃   CH₃

144

Actinomycin D
(Dactinomycin, cosmegen)

LE T/C 145, PS T/C >275 some cures
B1 T/C 203 (0.1 mg/kg), LL inactive
RO some cures

LE system, actinomycin D appeared to be synergistic with emetine and methotrexate but not with L-asparaginase or vincristine. With the L5178Y leukemia, a combination of actinomycin D and L- asparaginase showed a marked therapeutic potentiation. On the other hand, Chinese hamster cells in culture have been obtained with an acquired resistance to actinomycin D. Also actinomycin D was found to be cross-resistant to mithramycin, vincristine, vinblastine, daunomycin, and mitomycin C. These excellent studies with experimental tumor systems anticipated, in part, results of a recent clinical study involving alternate administration of adriamycin, vincristine, and actinomycin D in a series of patients with advanced and metastatic sarcomas incurable by surgical means.[87] The 20% objective response rate realized was about the same as that obtained by the use of either actinomycin D or adriamycin as single drugs. However, it should be noted that two patients, one with a fibrous histiocytoma and the other with a desmoid fibromatosis, were remarkably improved by this treatment.

Clinically actinomycin D has also been of value in the treatment of trophoblastic malignancies, testicular tumors, and soft tissue sarcomas. Indeed actinomycin D may be the most effective single agent available for testicular cancer.[246] With trophoblastic neoplasms, actinomycin D has proved as effective as methotrexate, and there appears to be no clinical cross-resistance between the two drugs. Individually actinomycin D, procarbazine, and vinblastine are all capable of producing objective responses ranging from 15% to 35% in patients with malignant melanoma. In combination, these three drugs have been found to yield an overall response rate of 38% with malignant melanoma.[295,367] Interestingly actinomycin D has also proved useful in the treatment of hypercalcemia arising from the abnormal (producing substances influencing body calcium levels) biosyntheses of certain tumors.

Present evidence suggests that actinomycin D forms a stable complex with DNA that interferes with DNA-dependent RNA syntheses. In fact, actinomycin D has been shown to inhibit the growth of DNA viruses, gram-positive bacteria, and mammalian cells both in culture and *in vivo*. Generally the growth of RNA viruses is not influenced by antinomycin D.[104] Circumstantial evidence that actinomycin D binds to DNA has been augmented by an X-ray crystallographic study of a complex formed between actinomycin D and deoxyguanosine. Interpretation of the X-ray data suggested that the phenoxazinone ring intercalates with guanine and a strong hydrogen bond is formed between the guanine 2-amino group and the carbonyl oxygen of the L-threonine unit. Hollstein and colleagues, using a circular dichroism method, suggest that CpG and GpC are the most favorable binding sites.[4a] Such a mechanism of action would suggest many possibilities for human toxicity. In practice, a variety of toxic reactions are encountered, ranging from dermatological and gastrointestinal to hematological.[155,246] Minor modification of the quinone phenoxazinone portion of actinomycin D may prove to be a most convenient avenue to obtaining better cancer chemotherapeutic agents of this type. Modest and colleagues[367] recently reported the preparation of several 7-substituted actinomycin D analogues and results of screening against the PS system. In this study, actinomycin D gave a PS T/C of 218, while the 7-nitro and 7-amino derivatives showed, respectively, T/C 254 and 264. Surely the renewed interest[273] in structural modification of actinomycin D will eventually yield substances with more favorable therapeutic indices and less serious toxicity.

A most unusual series of peptide anticancer antibiotics is represented by the bleomycins.[405,406] In the 1964–66 period, the Tokyo Institute of Microbial Chemistry group led by Umezawa, reported discovery of the bleomycins in *Streptomyces verticillus*.[166,407,408] The crude mixture of bleomycins was obtained as a bluish copper chelate. After the removal of the copper by complex formation with 8-hydroxyquinoline, the antitumor activity was retained. Careful separation of the antibiotic mixture led to eight bleomycins differing only in the amine portion of the thiazole amide.[391] The addition of amines, particularly diamines or triamines, during the fermentation procedure sup-

presses production of the usual bleomycins and favors formation of a bleomycin containing the added amine. By this means,
about 200 new bleomycins have been prepared.[406] The natural
bleomycin A$_2$ (**145**) is representative and is the principal (55-
70%) component of the bleomycin mixture originally used for
clinical studies in Japan.[405] Subsequent clinical studies with pure
bleomycin A$_2$ have indicated a greater degree of skin toxicity
than when the same amount is given as a component of the
mixture.

Bleomycin A$_2$ has proved to be a broad-spectrum antibiotic
and exhibits wide-ranging antitumor effects in experimental
animal systems, including Rous sarcoma virus, murine mam-
mary carcinomas, and the Ehrlich ascites carcinoma. But with
the LE leukemia, bleomycin A$_2$ is ineffective. In human
neoplastic disease, bleomycin A$_2$ has been found effective
against squamous-cell carcinoma, particularly of the penis and
the scrotum.[348] Generally a response rate of 20–40% has been
achieved with squamous-cell carcinoma at various sites. Objective responses have been obtained with 40–70% of patients with
testicular tumors and 30–60% of patients with lymphomas.[405] In
a recent study of stage III testicular neoplastic disease, the
complete response rate was improved by the use of a combination of bleomycin A$_2$ and vinblastine.[354] A related program,
including the use of methotrexate and radiation, has been
explored for bronchogenic carcinoma. The epidermoid carcinoma group responded best.[353]

Initially bleomycin A$_2$ is given clinically at a dose of approximately 2 mg/m^2 (0.0625 mg/kg) every fourth day for 6 weeks.
In Japan, bleomycin has been used intravenously or intramuscu-
larly twice a week at doses of 10–15 mg/m^2. With a total dose
greater than 200 mg/m^2, there is a great risk of fatal pulmonary
fibrosis.[405] Renal and skin toxicity are other areas of concern.
On the positive side, even high doses of bleomycin do not lead to
leukopenia or thrombocytopenia, and this lack of myelosuppressive toxicity indicates that bleomycin A$_2$ should be a very
useful addition to a combination formulation for cancer
chemotherapy.

145

Bleomycin A₂

LE inactive, PS T/C 150
B1 T/C 168, LL T/C 158 (18 mg/kg)

118
198
275
391
406

Apparently the antineoplastic effects of bleomycins can be attributed (in part) to their strand cleavage effects on DNA. They also inhibit the incorporation of thymidine into the DNA of intact cells and lead to inhibition of cell division, particularly during mitosis. This leads to daughter cells that enlarge, burst, and expire.[405] Thus the useful clinical activity, the intriguing biology, and the challenging chemistry offered by the bleomycins clearly warrant further structural modification and invite total synthetic efforts. Such study should provide insights into the design of structurally simpler drugs based on the unusual amino acids, β-lactam and dithiazole or the glucose and mannose portions of the molecule. At this time, it would seem that glycoside derivatives of certain small peptides would be a useful avenue to explore for antineoplastic activity.

A very nice illustration of an effective anticancer agent composed of only common amino acids is presented by neocarzinostatin (**146**). Here it becomes quite apparent that the proper sequencing of common amino acids will provide polypeptide or protein antineoplastic agents. The isolation of neocarzinostatin from *Streptomyces carzinostaticus* var. F-41 was achieved (1965) in Japan by Ishida and co-workers.[169] The 109 amino acid-unit protein structure (**146**) for neocarzinostatin was deduced by the Meienhofer group.[263] Meanwhile this small protein has been found to be active against gram-positive bacteria, a variety of murine tumor systems including SA,[278] and an ascites leukemia designated SN-36. The reaction of neocarzinostatin with succinic anhydride has led to the corresponding amide derivative, where all amino groups have been blocked. This succinamide was found to retain the antineoplastic activity, indicating that the free amino groups are not essential.[252]

Neocarzinostatin appears to inhibit DNA synthesis as well as degrading this biopolymer. As with bleomycin A_2, the net effect is on mitosis. Early Japanese reports suggest that neocarzinostatin might be useful in gastrointestinal cancer as well as in neoplastic disease of the bladder and the penis.[263] In the NCI's programs, neocarzinostatin has been under study for over 10 years, and toxicity investigations preliminary to clinical trial

252
263

Ala-Ala-Pro-Thr-Ala-Thr-Val-Thr-Pro-Ser-Ser-Gly-Leu-Ser-Asp-
Gly-Thr-Val-Val-Lys-Val-Ala-Gly-Ala-Gly-Leu-Gln-Ala-Gly-Thr-
$_{30}$
Ala-Tyr-Asp-Val-Gly-Gln-Cys-Ala-Ser-Val-Asn-Thr-Gly-Val-
Leu-Trp-Asn-Ser-Val-Thr-Ala-Ala-Gly-Ser-Ala-Cys-Asx-Pro-Ala-
Asn-Phe-Ser-Leu-Thr-Val-Arg-Arg-Ser-Phe-Glu-Gly-Phe-Leu-
$_{60}$
Phe-Asp-Gly-Thr-Arg-Trp-Gly-Thr-Val-Asx-Cys-Thr-Thr-Ala-
Ala-Cys-Gln-Val-Gly-Leu-Ser-Asp-Ala-Ala-Gly-Asp-Gly-Glu-
$_{90}$ $_{100}$
Pro-Gly-Val-Ala-Ile-Ser-Phe-Asn
$_{109}$

146

Neocarzinostatin

LE T/C 163, PS T/C > 200
LL T/C 124 (0.06 mg/kg)

have recently been summarized.[358] Investigations of small peptides, particularly those containing tryptophan, for antineoplastic properties have been under way in our laboratory for a number of years.[298] Results obtained to date leave no doubt that small polypeptides can be uncovered with anticancer activity. Now it appears obvious that structure/activity studies of neocarzinostatin and its total synthesis should be useful, and part of our present effort is devoted to these objectives. At least 10 antitumor antibiotics that appear to be proteins are known, and the latest additions are macracidmycin produced by *Streptomyces atrofaciens*[290] and renastacarcin from a *Streptomyces* sp.[357] Future sequential analyses of these protein antineoplastic agents should yield important information for structure/activity correlations. The antineoplastic carbohydrate biopolymers of fungal origin listed in Volume 2 represent another area of complex structural problems awaiting resolution.

The successful clinical application of L-asparaginase, mentioned in Chapter 1 and in more detail in Chapter 10, has stimulated the search for other enzymes capable of interfering with the metabolic requirements of neoplastic cells. Two advances in this direction are particularly noteworthy. Bertino and colleagues[54] have purified a folate-cleaving bacterial enzyme designated carboxypeptidase G_1 from *Pseudomonas stutzeri*. The enzyme was found to block the incorporation of deoxynucleosides into DNA and to have folate-depleting activity. The latter action arises from its hydrolysis action on the peptide bond of folic acid in both the reduced and the nonreduced forms. Most importantly, the enzyme completely inhibited growth of cell lines from LE, L5178Y, human lymphoblastoid 4265, and the Walker 256 carcinosarcoma, as well as showing *in vivo* activity against LE (27% life extension) and WA (89% life extension). Comparison studies with methotrexate indicate substantial differences in antineoplastic activity.

Other potentially important bacterial enzymes are the glutaminase–asparaginases from *Acinetobacter glutaminasificans* and *Pseudomonas aureofaciens*.[362] For certain neoplasms, the amino acid glutamine is necessary in quantities exceeding that for any other amino acid. Therefore certain neoplastic cells are more in need of glutamine than normal cells and a glutaminase would seem of some utility. Antineoplastic evaluation of the enzyme from *Acinetobacter g.* showed 90–100% inhibition of the asparaginase-resistant tumors EA, METHA sarcoma, and TAPER liver tumor in mice. At high dose levels, this enzyme was more effective than its *Pseudomonas a.* counterpart but less effective against experimental solid tumors.[362] The crude bacterial extracts known as *Corynebacterium parvum* vaccine and *Mycobacterium tuberculosis* vaccine (BCG) are now being considered for clinical trial by the NCI because of their ability to stimulate the immunological mechanism. From a bio-organic chemist's viewpoint, these are simply complex mixtures of biosynthetic products useful in cancer chemotherapy.

From a reading of this chapter, it should be perfectly clear that the lower plants are capable of synthesizing an astonishing structural variety of cancer chemotherapeutic agents. Based on the incredibly large number of such microorganisms believed to be available, this approach to clinically useful anticancer agents appears to be only at the bare beginning of exploration. So far, the Japanese, the Soviet Union, and the European programs directed at discovery of antineoplastic agents in the lower plants have been particularly productive and should provide an excellent model for future investigations, just as the very productive NCI program serves as a valuable model program for higher plants. With programs directed at plant and animal constituents (summarized in the following two chapters), the most pressing need is for greatly increased numbers of highly trained bio-organic chemists (and financial support) to do isolation and characterization studies and for research clinicians at the penultimate phase of drug development.

Marine Invertebrate and Other Lower Animal Biosynthetic Products

The species *Homo sapiens* of the mammalian order Primates includes all the races of true man. There is now evidence[343] provided by Leakey in Tanzania that true man has evolved and lived in Africa at least 3.75 million years. However, one can easily estimate that many of the lower animals, especially the marine invertebrates, have been in existence for at least 1–2 billion years. In this observer's judgment, biosynthetic evolutionary processes over such an incredibly long period would favor the development of very sophisticated chemical protective mechanisms that could be most useful in various areas of modern medical practice and specifically in cancer chemotherapy. In support of this view is the fact that invertebrates do not have a thymus system of immunological protection and therefore do not produce antibodies.[135] Obviously invertebrates must have developed mechanisms of intercellular control based on as yet unknown chemical regulation.

Invertebrates higher than the flatworm need a plasma for transporting metabolic and dissolved gas needs. Most have a pulsating organ except for members of the Annelida, which have a closed vascular arrangement. In the marine invertebrates, leukocytes function by encapsulating (phago-cytizing) foreign bodies and assist in wound healing. Thus phagocytosis is a primary defense system of invertebrates, presumably aided by relatively low molecular weight (non-protein) substances.[136] Again present evidence suggests that antibodies are not formed in invertebrates. Thus the biosyn-thetic compounds utilized in such control mechanisms should be of particular importance in the development of cancer chemotherapeutic agents. Another very important considera-tion is the observation that *cancer is virtually unknown among marine invertebrates.* So far, 10 species of bivalve molluscs from Australia, Japan, and the United States have been found with a neoplastic disease. In addition, benign epithelial neoplasm has been detected in one shrimp. These important facts are based on the excellent studies of Harshbarger.[136] Among terrestrial invertebrates, there have been reports of several probable cases of neoplastic disease in snails and of a transplantable invasive neoplasm in the fly *Drosophila melanogaster.*[134] Interestingly a transplantable invasive neoplasm of this organism is controlled by a single gene.[135]

Since there are over a million species of marine inverte-brates and about 1 million species just in the class Insecta of the arthropods, it seems very obvious that the invertebrates must have developed a sophisticated protection against neoplastic disease. Such considerations inspired our initiating a broad and systematic program beginning in 1965–66 to evaluate marine invertebrates[304] and arthropods[309] as sources of useful anti-cancer agents.

The potent physiological activity of marine animal con-stituents was well known to ancient man. One of the earliest recorded examples is hieroglyphics on the tomb of the Egyptian pharaoh Ti of approximately 2700 B.C. At that time, use of the poisonous puffer fish *Tetraodon stellatus* was already known. A fascinating description of the application of marine animal biosynthetic products in primitive medicine, including the use of stingray venom in Roman medicine of 29–79 A.D., has been summarized in the classic works of Halstead.[127]

In Chapter 2, it was mentioned that spongouridine (**39**) isolated from a sponge led eventually to synthesis of the clinically useful cytosine arabinoside (ara C). Before we leave this historical development of potential medicinal agents from marine invertebrates, another recent advance based on spongouridine should be mentioned. Recently the arabinoside of adenine[341] (**147**) has been found to show significant antiviral activity against herpes simplex and vaccina virus.[128]

From early 1950, there have been reports that extracts from starfish meal, the peanut worm *Bonellia fulginosa*, a clam, and certain sea cucumbers showed antineoplastic activity. By 1969, our broad geographic and taxonomic survey of marine animals for antineoplastic constituents had definitely established that these organisms should be a particularly useful source of potential cancer chemotherapeutic drugs.[304] Meanwhile we have continued to evaluate extracts of marine invertebrates on a worldwide basis, and by 1975, evaluation of about 8,000 extracts from 2,500 different species had led to the discovery of 250 species yielding extracts with confirmed-level activity in the National Cancer Institute (NCI) PS and/or KB screening systems. Almost half of these extracts have given PS T/C values of 150 or greater. We have located such marine invertebrate and vertebrate species from all of the marine animal phyla[243] except the Protozoa and some of the worm phyla, from which we have not yet obtained an adequate sampling.

Several years ago, Weinheimer began an analogous evaluation of marine animal extracts and has reported that of approximately 1,600 extracts, some 9% reached the confirmed level of activity in the NCI's exploratory screening program.[426] The University of Hawaii groups of Norton and Moore have also begun a study of marine animal antineoplastic constituents and have uncovered several species of coelenterates and annelids active against the Ehrlich ascites and PS experimental tumor systems.[283,284,333]

The marine animal program in our institute has now reached a reasonably mature level, where productivity begins to accelerate in terms of isolated and characterized anticancer constituents. In the past 10 years, we have been attempting to develop systematic methods[324] for isolating antineoplastic agents using bioassay techniques with the NCI's key tumor systems. As would be expected, marine animal extracts are considerably more challenging to separate than plant extracts, and development of simple methods has involved a protracted period of effort. One of these early studies involved the molluscs *Macrocallista nimbosa* and *Turbo stenogyrus* from respectively Florida and Taiwan. Only the marginally PS active amino acid taurine (**148**) was isolated.[320] With improvements in techniques, the next advance involved isolation and partial characterization of the major cytotoxic (PS *in vitro*) constituents of the Holothurioidea species *Actinopygia mauritiana* (from Hawaii), *Stichopus chloronotus* Brant (from Australia), and the Taiwan and Marshall Islands sea cucumber *Thelenota ananas* Jaeger.[311] We designated the three major cytotoxic constituents respectively actinostatin I, stichostatin I, and thelenostatin I. Preliminary structural investigation has indicated that all three substances are lanostane-type saponins related to holotoxin A. Attempts to elucidate the complete structures are now in progress. Interestingly a variety of such sea cucumbers (Echinodermata phylum) are marketed in Asia under the name Trepang and one of these, *Stichopus japonicus* Selenka, has been used for various medical treatments and as human food. Investigation of such sea cucumber toxins was already underway in 1929, and isolation of a saponin mixture was described in 1942.[311] In addition to antineoplastic activity, such saponins exhibit a variety of physiological properties, ranging from hemolytic to neurotoxic.

Present investigations in our institute range from the characterization of glycoprotein antineoplastic agents from the green sea urchin *Strongylocentrotus drobachiensis*[310] (Echinodermata) to the relatively low (less than 400) molecular weight and highly active (PS) constituents of the Australian and Indian Ocean mollusca *Aplysia angasi*[312a] and *Dolabella auricularia*.[321] While this volume was being completed, in January 1976, we succeeded in assigning novel structures **150**

341

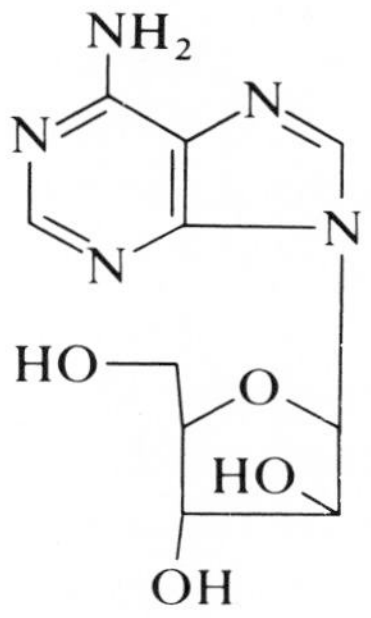

147

320

$$NH_2CH_2CH_2SO_3H$$

148

Taurine

PS T/C 131 (100 mg/kg)

and **150A** to the cytotoxic components aplysistatin[312a] and dolatriol 6-acetate[321] of the latter marine animals. From such stimulating results already at hand, eventual introduction of cancer chemotherapeutic drugs from marine animals seems a certainty.

Further support for the preceding conclusion is provided by initial results from the Norton, Moore, and Weinheimer programs. The stoichacetin isolated from the Tahitian sea anemone *Stoichactis kenti* has been shown capable of curing the murine Ehrlich ascites carcinoma.[283] Palytoxin, the toxic constituent of the Hawaiian Zoanthid *Palythoa toxica* (Coelenterata), has shown similar activity against the Ehrlich ascites carcinoma in mice but was only marginally active against the murine PS leukemia.[333] A cembranolide (**149**) reminiscent of the cytotoxic plant sesquiterpenes has been found to be the KB active constituent of four gorgonians of the *Pseudoplexaura* genus (collected in the Caribbean).[426] Crassin acetate (**149**), like taurine, showed only marginal activity against the PS leukemia, and neither of these initial results is in any way representative of the highly active marine animal constituents such as dolastatin now under study in our laboratory.

Concomitantly with the first systematic survey of marine animals for antineoplastic agents, we undertook an analogous study of terrestrial arthropods.[309] Antineoplastic evaluation (in the NCI's WA, PS, and/or KB screening procedures) of extracts from some 800 different arthropod species from the classes Insecta, Arachnida, Crustacea, and Myriapoda proved very encouraging. The yield of confirmed active extracts was approximately 4%, and for this reason, we have placed major emphasis upon development of the marine animal leads. However, this relatively small sample of arthropods did certainly confirm that the yield of confirmed active extracts would be substantially higher than that experienced with the lower plants and somewhat above that of the higher plants. Indeed the arthropods have been used since antiquity in primitive medical practice, and there is every reason to believe that certain arthropods will provide useful cancer chemotherapeutic agents.[309]

426

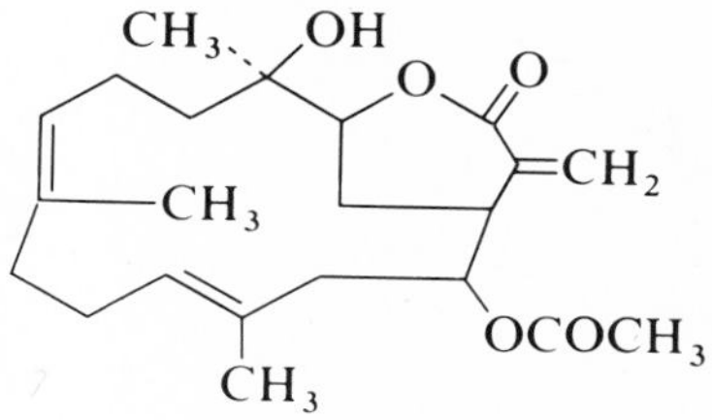

149

Crassin acetate

PS T/C 130 (50 mg/kg)

312*a*

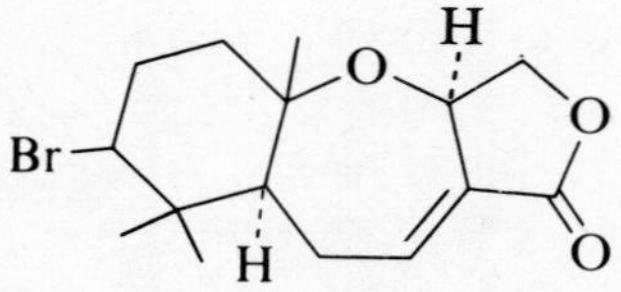

150

Aplysistatin

P388 ED$_{50}$ 2.7, KB ED$_{50}$ 2.4 μg/ml

321

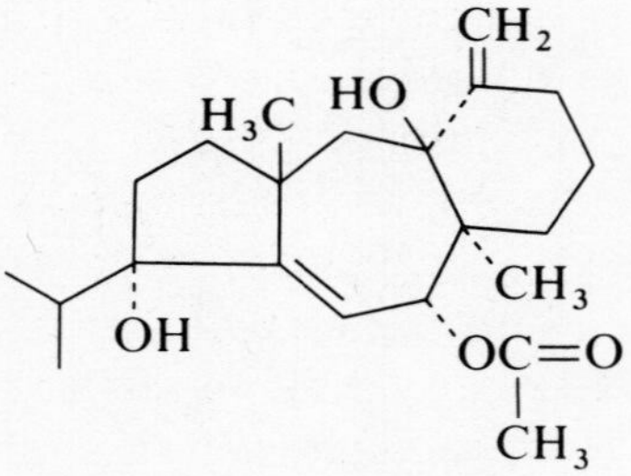

150A

Dolatriol 6-acetate

P388 ED$_{50}$ 13 μg/ml

Two of our group's early investigations in the arthropod field led to the first isolations of antineoplastic agents from such terrestrial invertebrates. Almost at the outset of our arthropod endeavors, the Asian butterfly *Catopsilia crocale* Cramer (Pieridae) gave an ethanol extract that reached the confirmed active stage in the WA tumor.[314] Eventually the antineoplastic constituent was located in the wings, and in order to have sufficient material for isolation by bioassay (in the Walker 256 carcinoma), it became necessary to employ up to 500 field collectors to obtain the necessary 250,000 members of this species. Subsequently the WA active biosynthetic product was found to be isoxanthopterin (**151**). Since the antineoplastic activity of pteridin **151** did not carry over to the PS system, we have been pursuing structural modifications of this substance. An analogous study of the Asian butterfly *Prioneris thestylis* Dbldy. indicates that the major antineoplastic constituent is simply isoguanine (**152**).[318]

Another Insecta species found of further interest soon after the program began was the stag beetle (Lucanidae family) *Allomyrina dichotomus* L. This beetle was obtained from trees in Taiwan, and an ethanol extract was found to exhibit confirmed-level activity against the WA carcinosarcoma. After considerable effort, the antineoplastic constituent was located in the legs of the female beetle.[319] Recently we have characterized the actual anticancer agent dichostatin as a protein of at least 106 amino acid units, and eventual elucidation of the complete structure should enhance the knowledge of polypeptide antineoplastic agents. Dichostatin was found to cause a 64% (at 3 mg/kg) inhibition of growth with the WA tumor and was only marginally active against the PS leukemia. Other such investigations among the arthropods are in progress, and it appears certain that a great number of cancer chemotherapeutic agents remain to be uncovered among the Arthropoda and other as yet unexplored lower animal phyla.

The most important conclusion to be reached from the coverage of this chapter is that the lower animals represent a virtually untapped but potentially very fruitful source of new

314

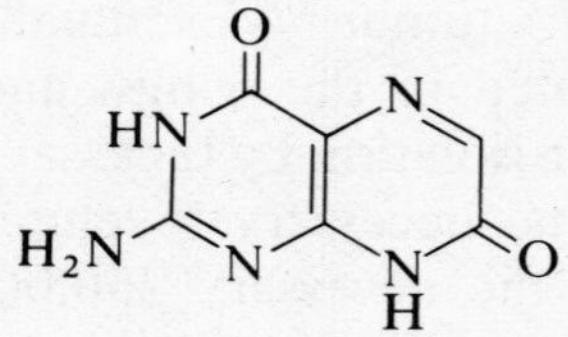

151

Isoxanthopterin

WA T/C 29 (90 mg/kg)

318

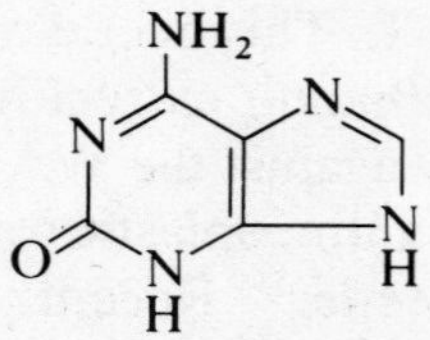

152

Isoguanine

CA active

cancer chemotherapeutic drugs. However, the challenges presented by this approach will continue to try the chemist's patience and that of their philanthropic and granting agency supporters. Given sufficient financial support and time, the lower animals will prove to be a particularly good source of unusual and valuable drugs for cancer chemotherapy.

Chapter 10

Marine Vertebrate and Other Higher Animal Biosynthetic Products

Neoplastic disease and its fatal consequences is an all-too-frequent occurrence among many species of higher animals. But cancer is relatively rare among many types of lower vertebrates, and even the higher vertebrates must have elaborately sophisticated biosynthetic products that normally prevent transgression by neoplastic invasion. In the lower vertebrates, known cases of cancer can be summarized as follows. Among the marine and fresh-water fish (superclass Pisces, phylum Chordata, subphylum Vertebrata), Harshbarger at the Smithsonian Institution has recorded a large number of species with neoplasms, including epizootic hepatomas in a population of Atlantic hagfish, a metastatic melanoma in a single lamprey, and neoplasms in some five families of Chondrichthyes, including cat sharks, requiem sharks, ratfish, and skates.[134] Interestingly neoplastic disease among such marine vertebrates is generally of the mesenchymal type, unlike that of human cancer.[260]

The occurrence of cancer in various amphibians (superclass Tetrapoda, class Amphibia) has been well established, particularly the renal adenocarcinoma of the leopard frogs initiated by a herpes virus. In toads of the genus *Bufo*, a few tumors have been recorded but seem to be of the type initiated by bacterial invasion. For example, *B. regularis* has been found with a soft lump posterior to the left eye that on pathological examination, proved to be a granuloma containing very small, gram-positive, rod-shaped bacteria.[137] Similarly a specimen of *B. marinus* has been found with a lymphatic cyst on its head, a specimen of *B. boreas* with a fibroma, a specimen of *B. americanus* with randomly scattered lesions probably due to parasites, and a specimen of *B. arenarum* with an infectious granuloma.[137]

Among the marine reptiles (superclass Tetrapoda, class Reptilia), a neoplasm has been found on one specimen of a green sea turtle. Among terrestrial reptiles, a number are known to incur neoplastic disease, such as lymphosarcoma in the Egyptian cobra *Naja naja*, in the river Jack *Bitis nasicornis*, and in the hognose snake *Heterodon platyrhinos*. The timber rattlesnake, *Crotalus horridus horridus*, has been found with widespread neoplastic disease, including of the lungs, the liver, the heart, and the kidneys. The first example of a hematopoietic neoplasm in a lacertilian—namely, the lizard *Hydrosaurus amboinensis*—is now known.[136] In addition, the Schmidt Ruppin strain of Rous sarcoma virus has been found oncogenic to two lizards, a turtle, and the sand boa, *Eryx tataricus*. Among mammals (superclass Tetrapoda, class Mammalia), the occurrence of cancer in a great many varieties is ubiquitous in animals ranging from various rodents to cats, dogs, swine, cattle, horses, monkeys, gibbons, and finally man.

For reasons already outlined in the preceding chapter, our group undertook (1966) the first systematic investigation of marine vertebrates for antineoplastic constituents.[304] The results of this effort have been exceptionally rewarding, and so far 57 species of fish have been uncovered that give extracts reaching the confirmed active stage in the National Cancer Institute (NCI) PS and/or KB exploratory screen. Also in the phylum Chordata we have found a number of tunicates (class Larvacea) and ascidians (class Ascidiacea) with antineoplastic constituents. The isolation and characterization of the actual antineoplastic components have been quite challenging, but several of these problems are nearing completion. Our experience with the hammerhead shark, *Sphyrna lewini*, has been typical. Here the PS active constituent has been located in the blood and the body fluids as well as in the muscle and the liver. The active agent was found to be a high molecular weight ($>40 \times 10^6$) glycoprotein, quite soluble in water.[318] Analogous investigations of other shark species are in progress in our institute, and the eventual results should be of particular interest. Most species of the 200 or more known sharks have not been found with cancer. In related studies from a Moscow medical institute, a protamine fraction (called stellin) from sturgeon milt has been shown to inhibit growth of some murine tumor systems.[292] For other appraisals of the potential of marine invertebrates and vertebrates in producing medicinally valuable substances, the reader is referred to recent reviews by Baslow,[19] Djerassi,[84] and Scheuer.[361] Additionally we are in the process of preparing a compilation of all known marine animal biosynthetic products, which may be available within the year.[318]

Applications of amphibian extracts, particularly from toads of the genus *Bufo* (Bufonidae family), in primitive medical treatment have been known for at least several millennia.[307] The use of toad venom as well as that from certain frogs for the tips of blow-pipe darts represents another long-standing utilization of amphibian biosynthetic products. Knowledge of the toxic properties of certain salamander components must also date back to antiquity. However, the toad venoms have been most prominently mentioned in early medical treatments. Especially significant have been applications of venom from *B. bufo gargarizans*, which is used in the Chinese medicinal preparation Ch'an Su.[183] In a 1596 Chinese medical treatise, Ch'an Su was described in the treatment of canker sores (known to be caused by a herpes virus), local inflammation, toothache, and gum hemorrhage.[261] In June 1974, while in the People's Republic of China, this writer was very interested to see specimens of *B. bufo gargarizans* prominently exhibited in medical collections and to learn of current applications of Ch'an Su in traditional medical treatment, primarily based on its anesthetic, anti-inflammatory, and cardiac effects. In the latter respect, it is interesting to recall that several European pharmacopoeias published between 1672 and 1702 highly recommended powdered toad skin for congestive heart failure. However, the introduction of *digitalis* in 1775, by the Scottish physician Withering, probably caused abandonment of the more difficultly obtained toad venom for cardiac problems. In another medical area, a 15th-century European medical text described the use of toad extract in the treatment of difficult breathing.[58]

Serious chemical investigation of toad venom constituents was under way with the beginning of this century, and by the later 1940's, structures were known for some of the more common steroidal bufadienolide constituents, such as bufalin (**153**) and resibufogenin (**154**). Now almost 50 such bufadienolides have been characterized from various toad venoms, and a majority of these have been found in Ch'an Su.[196] Meanwhile pharmacological studies of several pure bufadienolides have revealed, for example, that bufalin (**153**) has cardiac activity about equal to that of digitoxigenin and a local anesthetic potency on the rabbit cornea approximately 90 times that of cocaine.[307] Other bufadienolides from toad venom, such as cinobufagin, are also known to have substantial local anesthetic effects. In general, most bufadienolides act directly on smooth muscles and are vasoconstrictors.[58] Several members of this series have been considered for clinical trial as substitutes for certain of the cardenolides and some may someday find such application. Resibufogenin (**154**) has been successfully introduced into clinical practice in Japan as a respiratory stimulant.

Based on a 1948 report by Haynes,[150] the possibility that certain α,β-unsaturated lactones might inhibit cell growth stimulated this writer to initiate a program in 1957 directed at obtaining sufficient amounts of the toad venom constituents for antineoplastic evaluation. At that time, the most workable solution to this problem seemed to be the development of total syntheses of the toad venom bufadienolides. Up to the present writing, we have completed the first total syntheses for 14 of the bufadienolide toad venom constituents.[183] Bufadienolides **153**

145
168
181
196

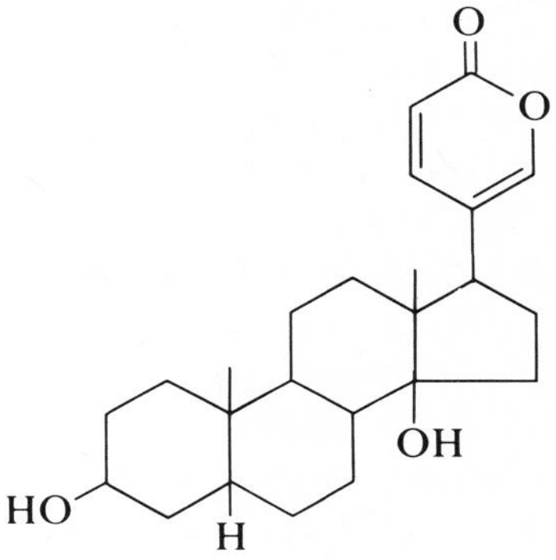

153

Bufalin

P338 ED$_{50}$ 20, KB <0.1 μg/ml

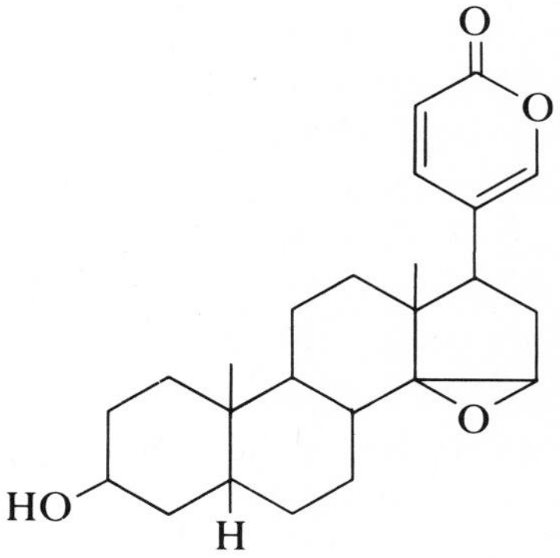

154

Resibufogenin

P388 ED$_{50}$ 15, KB 0.34 μg/ml

and **154** were the first to be obtained by synthesis[181,317] and are now being assessed for *in vivo* antineoplastic activity. So far, marinobufagin (**155**), isolated from the American toad *B. marinus* and now available by synthesis,[316] has received the most detailed antineoplastic evaluation. In this collaborative study with the NCI, marinobufagin (**155**) was found to display the usual cytotoxic activity in the KB system and to inhibit the growth of the Ehrlich ascites carcinoma with about a 30% cure rate, but it was inactive in the LE and PS systems.[315] Evaluation against several experimental solid tumors is in progress. A considerable amount of further work will be necessary to evaluate amphibian constituents properly as potential cancer chemotherapeutic agents. The little information now at hand is about the toad genus *Bufo*, and very little is known about members of other genera and, of course, the frogs and salamanders. Also structural modification of the bufadienolides has barely begun.

The venom constituents of terrestrial and marine reptiles represent another avenue to possible new antineoplastic agents that has received only preliminary study. However, the snake venoms are generally very complex mixtures of polypeptides and proteins, so isolation of individual constituents in pure form is generally a very difficult task. The most advanced achievement of possible interest in the development of antineoplastic agents has been isolation of the cytotoxic component known as cytotoxin II from cobra venom.[390] The complete structure of cytotoxin II has been found to be a 60-amino-acid-unit polypeptide with four disulfide bridges. A recent study by Tu[402] of various snake venoms and derived fractions against the KB and Yoshida sarcoma cell lines indicated that venoms from the Crotalidae, the Elapidae, and the Viperidae caused lysis of both neoplastic cell lines as well as of normal peritoneal cells from the rat. Unfortunately these results suggested that snake venoms can be about equally effective in inhibiting growth of both tumor and normal cells. Interestingly venoms from the marine (sea snakes) Hydrophiidae did not lyse the neoplastic cells. With the paucity of information now available about the antineoplastic

316

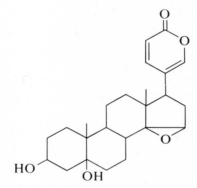

155

Marinobufagin

KB 0.086 μg/ml, EA T/C 155 (1.25 mg/kg)
and some cures, LE and PS inactive

components of reptiles, it is still too early to assess the future prospects for this category of animal biosynthetic products. But the wide-ranging pharmacological activity of reptile venoms does suggest that some, and/or their synthetic modifications, will eventually find a place in medicine.

The higher animals synthesize a great variety of simple to exceedingly complex substances with a dazzling spectrum of biological properties. Of course, those biosynthetic products that must normally control the advance of neoplastic changes would be of most interest from the viewpoint of the development of cancer chemotherapeutic drugs. A considerable number of leads have been recorded involving, for example, the antineoplastic effects of human protein hormones, such as parathyroid, glucagon, insulin, and thymus gland fractions; enzymes such as fibrinolysin; tissue extracts of spleen, liver, kidney, testicle, muscle, and placenta; and certain protamines and histones. Early work concerned with these possibilities has been nicely reviewed by Neuss, Gorman, and Johnson.[277] Recent developments in the chemistry of human polypeptide and protein hormones has been reviewed in another reference work by this author.[300] A very limited search for antineoplastic constituents in human tissue has been continuing, and one of the more interesting advances concerns the isolation of a cytotoxic fraction from human spleen.[249] Another cytotoxic fraction has been isolated from the plasma membranes obtained from the regional lymph nodes of CBA mice.[383] Attempts are presently being made to utilize the possible cancer-inhibiting effects of vitamins A and C.[299] Unfortunately a phase I clinical study of vitamin A ethylamide did not uncover any antineoplastic effects.[376]

The most successful higher animal antineoplastic constituent with respect to clinical utility has been the enzyme L-asparaginase originally isolated from guinea pig serum. In 1953, Kidd[191] reported that murine lymphoma was inhibited by guinea pig serum, and in 1961, Broome[40,41] established that the antineoplastic constituent was an L-asparaginase. Later it was found that only serum from species of the super family Cavioidea have an L-asparaginase with the proper antineoplastic activity. Among the plants only *Escherichia coli* B, *Serratia marcescens*, and the more potent source *Erwinia carotovora* have been found to produce an L-asparaginase with appropriate antitumor activity.[49,385]

Of particular importance in evaluation of the use of BCG vaccine from *Mycobacterium tuberculosis* (see Chapter 8) in cancer therapy is the report by Subba Reddy and co-workers[385] that L-asparagine amidohydrolases from the $H_{37} R_A$ strain of this microorganism were found to be very effective in inhibiting the growth of the Yoshida ascites sarcoma in rats. A second L-asparaginase from the same strain did not exhibit this antineoplastic activity, and the single L-asparaginase from another strain of *M. tuberculosis* was also inactive. The present commercial source of L-asparaginase for clinical use is from *E. Coli* B.[236]

In neoplastic cells, L-asparaginase inhibits protein synthesis dependent upon asparagine and eventually inhibits the synthesis of DNA and RNA. A substantial number (50) of murine neoplasms, three rat neoplasms, and the canine lymphosarcoma are inhibited by L-asparaginase.[49] Only the Rauscher leukemia virus of the mouse is susceptible to L-asparaginase; the other virus-induced leukemias are not sensitive to this enzyme treatment.

Clinically L-asparaginase has been used with the greatest success in the treatment of acute lymphocytic leukemia in children. A 35–60% complete remission rate has been realized, but the remissions have been fairly short probably because of the survival and proliferation of neoplastic cells with enough asparagine synthetase activity to replace the depleted exogenous asparagine.[247] Human toxic reactions to L-asparaginase are usually manageable and reversible. As would be expected, ammonia from the enzymatic cleavage of the asparagine amide leads to evaluated blood ammonia levels. Of particular importance is the observation that L-asparaginase is nearly free of gastrointestinal and myelosuppressive toxicity.[247] In general, the toxic effects involve the liver, occasional CNS depression or hyperexcitation, reduced blood-clotting ability, hypocholesterolemia, and the results of hypersensitivity. Interestingly man and cattle have a relatively high incidence of lymphomas, and both species have either a low level or lack detectable L-asparaginase. Unfortunately initial clinical trials of L-asparaginase in the treatment of human lyphomas as well as a series of solid tumors did not give any encouraging results.

Thus the goal of identifying a higher animal biosynthetic product with great selectivity for neoplastic cells and minimal toxicity to normal cells is still unrealized but should remain a great stimulus to further research. Indeed this observer's most urgent wish is that many of the approaches outlined in this volume will inspire increased research directed at uncovering clinically useful biosynthetic products for eventual control and cure of human cancer.

References

1. E. M. Acton, A. N. Fujiwara, and D. W. Henry. *J. Med. Chem.* *17*, 659 (1974).
2. A. B. Adolphe, E. D. Glasofer, W. M. Troetel, J. Ziegenfuss, J. E. Stambaugh, A. J. Weiss, and R. W. Manthei. *Cancer Chemother. Rep.* Pt 1, *59*, 547 (1975).
3. V. N. Aiyar and F. C. Chang. *J. Org. Chem. 40*, 2384 (1975).
4. A. Akahori, F. Yasuda, M. Ando, K. Hori, and T. Okanishi. *Chem. Pharm. Bull. (Tokyo) 20*, 1150 (1972).
4a. F. S. Allen, R. P. Moen, and U. Hollstein. *J. Amer. Chem. Soc. 98*, 864 (1976).
5. M. Ando, G. Büchi, and T. Ohnuma. *J. Amer. Chem. Soc. 97*, 6880 (1975).
6. R. Angiuli, E. Foresti, L. Riva di Sanseverino, N. W. Isaacs, O. Kennard, W. D. S. Motherwell, D. L. Wampler, and F. Arcamone. *Nature New Biol. 234*, 78 (1971).
7. F. J. Antosz, D. B. Nelson, D. L. Herald, Jr., and M. E. Munk. *J. Amer. Chem. Soc. 92*, 4933 (1970).
8. F. Arcamone, W. Barbieri, G. Franceschi, and S. Penco. *Chim. Ind. (Milan) 51*, 834 (1969).
9. F. Arcamone, G. Cassinelli, G. Franceschi, P. Orezzi, and R. Mondelli. *Tetrahedron Lett.*, 3353 (1968).
10. F. Arcamone, S. Penco, and A. Vigevani. *Cancer Chemother. Rep.* Pt 3, *6*, 123 (1975).
11. B. H. Arison and J. L. Beck. *Tetrahedron 29*, 2743 (1973).
12. H. R. Arthur, W. H. Hui, and Y. L. Ng. *Chem. Ind. (London)*, 1514 (1958).
13. J. Auerbach, T. Ipaktchi, and S. M. Weinreb. *Tetrahedron Lett.*, 4561 (1973).
14. J. Auerback and S. M. Weinreb. *J. Amer. Chem. Soc. 94*, 7172 (1972).
14a. D. Avnir, A. Grauer, D. Dinur, and J. Blum. *Tetrahedron 31*, 2457 (1975).
15. N. R. Bachur. *Biochem. Pharmacol.* 207, Supplement No. 2 (1974).
16. G. P. Bakhaeva, Y. A. Berlin, E. F. Boldyreva, O. A. Chuprunova, M. N. Kolosov, V. W. Soifer, T. E. Vasiljeva, and I. V. Yartseva. *Tetrahedron Lett.*, 3595 (1968).
17. D. Baltimore. *Nature 226*, 1209 (1970).
18. S. Barnes. *Smithsonian 5*, 50 (1975).
19. M. H. Baslow. *Marine Pharmacology*. The Williams and Wilkins Co., Baltimore, 1969.
20. F. J. Baur. *J. Amer. Oil Chem. Soc. 52*, 263 (1975).
21. J. R. Beck, R. Kwok, R. N. Booher, A. C. Brown, L. E. Patterson, P. Pranc, B. Rockey, and A. Pohland. *J. Amer. Chem. Soc. 90*, 4706 (1968).
22. F. F. Becker, Ed. "Cancer—A Comprehensive Treatise," Vol. 2, *Etiology, Viral Carcinogenesis*. Plenum Publishing Corp., New York, 1975.

23.   R. S. Benjamin, P. H. Wiernik, and N. R. Bachur. *Med. Ped. Oncol. 1*, 63 (1975).

24.   R. Bentley . *Pharm. J. Trans. 3*, 456 (1861).

25.   W. Bergmann and D. C. Burke. *J. Org. Chem. 20*, 1501 (1955).

26.   W. Bergmann and R. J. Feeney. *J. Amer. Chem. Soc. 72*, 2809 (1950).

27.   J. Bernard, J. Marie, J. Salet, and C. Cruciani. *Bull. Mem. Soc. Med. Hopitaux 16*, 621 (1951).

28.   B. K. Bhuyan. *Appl. Microbiol. 10*, 302 (1962).

29.   E. Bianchi and J. R. Cole. *J. Pharm. Sci. 58*, 589 (1969).

30.   J. H. Birkinshaw, A. Bracken, E. N. Morgan, and H. Raistrick. *Biochem. J. 43*, 216 (1948).

31.   J. H. Birkinshaw, H. Raistrick, and D. J. Ross. *Biochem. J. 50*, 630 (1952).

32.   W. A. Bleyer, S. A. Frisby, and V. T. Oliverio. *Biochem. Pharmacol. 24*, 633 (1975).

33.   J. B. Block, A. A. Serpick, W. Miller, and P. H. Wiernik. *Cancer Chemother. Rep.* Pt 2, *4*, 27 (1974).

33a. G. Bonadonna, E. Brusamolino, P. Valagussa, A. Rossi, L. Brugnatelli, C. Brambilla, M. De Lena, G. Tancini, E. Bajetta, R. Musumeci, and U. Veronesi. *New Eng. J. Med. 294*, 406 (1976).

34.   G. Bonadonna, R. Zucali, S. Monfardini, M. De Lena, and C. Uslenghi. *Cancer 36*, 252 (1975).

35.   M. G. Brazhnikova, V. B. Zbarsky, V. I. Ponomarenko, and N. P. Potapova. *J. Antibiot. (Tokyo) 27*, 254 (1974).

36.   British 974,541 (Upjohn Co.) Nov. 4, 1964; U.S. Appl. Oct. 26, 1961 [*Chem. Abstr. 62*, 5855d (1965)].

37.   British National Lymphoma Investigation (Report from). *Brit. Med. J. 3*, 413 (1975).

38.   H. Brockmann. *Fortschr. Chem. Org. Naturst. 18*, 1 (1960).

39.   J. E. Brody in *New York Times*, Dec. 3, 1975, pp. 1 and 71.

40.   J. D. Broome. *J. Exp. Med. 118*, 99 and 121 (1963).

41.   J. D. Broome. *Nature 191*, 1114 (1961).

42.   G. Büchi, K-C. Luk, and P. M. Müller. *J. Org. Chem. 40*, 3458 (1975).

43.   J. H. Burchenal. *Cancer 35*, 1121 (1975).

44.   B. F. Cain, G. J. Atwell, and R. N. Seelye. *J. Med. Chem. 14*, 311 (1971).

45.   M. Calvin. *Naturwissenschaften 62*, 405 (1975).

46.   *Cancer Chemother. Rep.* Pt 3, *6* (1975).

47.   *Cancer Chemother. Rep.* No. 1, *58* (1974).

48.   L. Canonica, B. Rindone, E. Santaniello, and C. Scolastico. *Tetrahedron 28*, 4395 (1972).

49.   R. L. Capizzi and R. E. Handschumacher. "Asparaginase," Section XIII, in *Cancer Medicine*, Ed. by J. F. Holland and E. Frei, III. Lea and Febiger, Philadelphia, 1973, p. 850.

50.   S. K. Carter. *U.S. Nat'l. Cancer Inst. Monographs 40*, 31 (1974).

51.   S. K. Carter. *Cancer 30*, 1402 (1972).

52.   S. K. Carter and R. L. Comis. *Cancer Treat. Rev.*, in press.

53.   S. K. Carter and L. M. Kershner. *Pharmacy Times*, 56 (1975).

54.   B. A. Chabner, P. L. Chellow, and J. R. Bertino. *Cancer Res. 32*, 2114 (1972).

55.   E. Chain, H. W. Florey, A. D. Gardner, N. G. Heatley, M. A. Jennings, J. Orr-Ewing, and A. G. Sanders. *Lancet 2*, 226 (1940).

56. B. C. Challis and C. D. Bartlett. *Nature 254*, 532 (1975).
57. C-J. Chang, H. G. Floss, P. Soong, and C-T. Chang. *J. Antibiot. (Tokyo) 28*, 156 (1975).
58. K. K. Chen and A. Kovaříková. *J. Pharm. Sci. 56*, 1535 (1967).
59. H. C. Chopa and W. F. Feller. *Tex. Rep. Biol. Med. 27*, 945 (1969).
60. Cold Spring Harbor Symposia on Quantitative Biology, Vol. 39, "Tumor Viruses." Cold Spring Harbor Laboratory, 1975.
61. M. da Consolação, F. Linardi, M. M. de Oliveira, and M. R. P. Sampaio. *J. Med. Chem. 18*, 1159 (1975).
62. J. W. Cook and J. D. Loudon. "Colchicine," Chapter X, in *The Alkaloids, Chemistry and Physiology*, Vol. 2, Ed. by R. H. F. Manske and H. L. Holmes. Academic Press, New York, 1952, p. 261.
63. R. L. Comis and S. K. Carter. *Cancer Treat. Rev.*, in press.
64. G. A. Cordell. *Lloydia 37*, 219 (1974).
65. E. J. Corey, D. N. Crouse, and J. E. Anderson. *J. Org. Chem. 40*, 2140 (1975).
66. E. J. Corey and B. B. Snider. *J. Amer. Chem. Soc. 94*, 2549 (1972).
67. P. J. Creaven, M. H. Cohen, O. S. Selawry, F. Tejada, and L. E. Broder. *Cancer Chemother. Rep.* Pt 1, *59*, 1001 (1975).
68. L. Crombie, M. L. Games, and D. L. Pointer. *J. Chem. Soc.* (C), 1347 (1968).
69. C. C. J. Culvenor. *J. Pharm. Sci. 57*, 1112 (1968).
70. M. Curcumelli-Redostamo and M. Kulka in *The Alkaloids*, Vol. 9, Ed. by R. H. F. Manske. Academic Press, New York, 1967, p. 133.
71. S. J. Cutler, M. H. Myers, and S. B. Green. *New Eng. J. Med.*, *293*, 122 (1975).
72. J. H. Cutts. *Proc. Am. Assoc. Cancer Res. 2*, 289 (1958).
73. J. H. Cutts, C. T. Beer, and R. L. Noble. *Cancer Res. 20*, 1023 (1960).
74. J. H. Cutts, C. T. Beer, and R. L. Noble. *Rev. Can. Biol. 16*, 487 (1957).
75. L. K. Dalton, S. Demerac, B. C. Elmes, J. W. Loder, J. M. Swan, and T. Teitei. *Aust. J. Chem. 20*, 2715 (1967).
76. K. R. Darnall, L. B. Townsend, and R. K. Robins. *Proc. Nat. Acad. Sci. 57*, 548 (1967).
77. T. Davis. *Med. J. Australia 2*, 228 (1975).
78. N. E. Day. *Cancer Res. 35*, 3304 (1975).
79. V. T. De Vita and P. S. Schein. *New Eng. J. Med. 288*, 998 (1973).
80. V. De Vita, A. Serpick, and P. Carbone. *Ann. Intern. Med. 73*, 881 (1970).
81. V. T. De Vita, Jr., R. C. Young, and G. P. Canellos. *Cancer 35*, 98 (1975).
82. A. DiMarco, M. Gaetani, L. Dorigotti, M. Soldati, and O. Bellini. *Cancer Chemother. Rep. 38*, 31 (1964).
83. A. DiMarco, M. Gaetani, and B. Scarpinato. *Cancer Chemother. Rep. 53*, 33 (1969).
84. C. Djerassi. *Pure Appl. Chem. 41*, 113 (1975).
85. R. W. Doskotch and F. S. El-Feraly. *J. Pharm. Sci. 58*, 877 (1969).
86. R. W. Doskotch, S. L. Keely, Jr., and C. D. Hufford. *J.C.S. Chem. Commun.*, 1137 (1972).
87. H. O. Douglass, Jr. and C. Karakousis. *Cancer Chemother. Rep.* Pt 1, *59*, 1035 (1975).
88. J. Druey. *Angew. Chem. 72*, 677 (1960).
89. L. R. Duvall. *Cancer Chemother. Rep. 7*, 86 (1960).

90. C. N. Eaton, G. H. Denny, Jr., M. A. Ryder, M. G. Ly, and R. D. Babson. *J. Med. Chem. 16*, 289 (1973).
91. B. Ebbell. *The Papyrus Ebers.* Oxford Univ. Press, London, 1937.
92. T. E. Eble and F. R. Hanson. *Antibiot. Chemother. 1*, 54 (1951).
93. S. Eckhardt, E. Döbrentey, and I. Bodrogi. *Chemotherapy 21*, 248 (1975).
94. K. M. Endicott. *J. Nat. Cancer Inst. 19*, 275 (1957).
94*a*. J. E. Enstrom. *Cancer 36*, 825 (1975).
94*b*. L. F. Fajardo and A. Lee. *Cancer 36*, 904 (1975).
95. S. Farber. *Amer. J. Pathol. 31*, 583 (1955).
96. S. Farber, C. Maddock, and M. Swaffield. *Proc. Am. Assoc. Cancer Res. 2*, 104 (1956).
97. S. Farber, R. Toch, E. M. Sears, and D. Pinkel. "Advances in Chemotherapy of Cancer in Man," in *Advances in Cancer Research*, Vol. 4, Ed. by J. P. Greenstein and A. Haddow. Academic Press, New York, 1956, p. 1.
98. L. N. Ferguson. *Chem. Soc. Rev. 4*, 289 (1975).
99. L. F. Fieser. *The Scientific Method.* Reinhold Publishing Corp., New York, 1964.
100. B. Fisher, P. Carbone, S. G. Economou, R. Frelick, A. Glass, H. Lerner, C. Redmond, M. Zelen, P. Band, D. L. Katrych, N. Wolmark, and E. R. Fisher. *New Eng. J. Med. 292*, 117 (1975).
101. A. Fleming. *Brit. J. Exp. Pathol. 10*, 226 (1929).
102. E. Frei. *New Eng. J. Med. 293*, 146 (1975).
103. E. Frei, N. Jaffe, M. H. N. Tattersall, S. Pitman, and L. Parker. *New Eng. J. Med. 292*, 846 (1975).
104. P. A. Friedman and A. Cerami. "Actinomycin," Section XIII, in *Cancer Medicine*, Ed. by J. F. Holland and E. Frei, III. Lea and Febiger, Philadelphia, 1973, p. 835.
105. A. N. Fujiwara, E. M. Acton, and D. W. Henry. *J. Med. Chem. 17*, 392 (1974).
106. R. E. Gallagher and R. C. Gallo. *Science 187*, 350 (1975).
107. G. F. Gause *et al. Antibiotiki 20*, 389 (1975).
108. G. F. Gause, M. G. Brazhnikova, and V. A. Shorin. *Cancer Chemother. Rep.* Pt 1, *58*, 255 (1974).
109. G. F. Gause, M. A. Sveshikova, R. S. Ukholina, G. V. Gavrilina, V. A. Filicheva, and E. G. Gladkikh. *Antibiotiki 18*, 675 (1973).
110. C. F. Geiser and J. W. Mitus. *Cancer Chemother. Rep.* Pt 1, *59*, 385 (1975).
111. E. Gellert and R. Rudzats. *J. Med. Chem. 7*, 361 (1964).
112. R. E. Gerner, H. Kitamura, and G. E. Moore. *Oncology 31*, 31 (1975).
113. M. Ghione. *Cancer Chemother. Rep.* Pt 3, *6*, 83 (1975).
114. P. G. Gill and J. Ludbrook. *Med. J. Australia 2*, 226 (1975).
115. J. P. Gillespie, L. D. Amoros, and F. R. Stermitz. *J. Org. Chem. 39*, 3239 (1974).
116. A. Goldin. *Chemtech.*, 424 (1972).
117. A. Goldin and S. K. Carter. "Screening and Evaluation of Antitumor Agents," Section XII, in *Cancer Medicine*, Ed. by J. F. Holland and E. Frei, III. Lea and Febiger, Philadelphia, 1973, p. 605.
118. A. Goldin and R. K. Johnson. *Cancer Chemother. Rep.* Pt 1, *58*, 63 (1974).
119. M. A. Goldsmith and S. K. Carter. *Cancer 33*, 1 (1974).
120. K. W. Gopinath, J. M. Kohli, M. S. Y. Khan, and A. R. Kidwai. *Indian J. Chem. 1*, 99 (1968).

121. J. A. Gottlieb and D. C. Hill, Jr. *New Eng. J. Med. 290*, 193 (1974).

122. J. A. Gottlieb, S. E. Rivkin, S. C. Spigel, B. Hoogstraten, R. M. O'Bryan, F. C. Delaney, and A. Singhakowinta. *Cancer 33*, 519 (1974).

123. T. R. Govindachari. "Tylophora Alkaloids," Chapter 13, in *The Alkaloids*, Vol. 9, Ed. by R. H. F. Manske. Academic Press, New York, 1967, p. 517.

124. C. D. Haagensen. *Amer. J. Cancer 18*, 42 (1933).

125. J. F. Halazun, H. R. Wagner, J. F. Gaeta, and L. F. Sinks. *Cancer 33*, 545 (1974).

126. T. J. Haley. *J. Pharm. Sci. 64*, 1435 (1975).

127. R. W. Halstead. "Poisonous and Venomous Marine Animals of the World," 1, 2. U.S. Government Printing Office, Washington, D.C., 1965, 1967.

128. S. Hanessian. *J. Med. Chem. 16*, 291 (1973).

129. L. J. Haňka, D. G. Martin, and G. L. Neil. *Cancer Chemother. Rep.* Pt 1, *57*, 141 (1973).

130. J. R. Hanson. "Diterpenoids," Chapter III, in *Terpenoids and Steroids*, Vol. 1. The Chemical Society, London, 1971, p. 124.

131. J. R. Hanson. "The Biosynthesis of the Diterpenes," in *Progress in the Chemistry of Organic Natural Products*, Vol. 29, Ed. by W. Herz, H. Grisebach, and G. W. Kirby. Springer-Verlag, New York, 1971, p. 395.

132. E. Hanssen and M. Jung. *Pure Appl. Chem. 35*, 239 (1973).

133. E. Härri, W. Loeffler, H. P. Sigg, H. Stamelin, C. Stoll, C. Tamm, and D. Wiesinger. *Helv. Chim. Acta 45*, 839 (1962).

134. J. C. Harshbarger (Smithsonian Institution), private communication, 1975.

135. J. C. Harshbarger. *Fed. Proc. 32*, 2224 (1973).

136. J. C. Harshbarger and C. J. Dawe. "Hematopoietic Neoplasms in Invertebrate and Poikilothermic Vertebrate Animals," in *Unifying Concepts of Leukemia*, Bibl. haemat., No. 39, Ed. by R. M. Dutcher and L. Chieco-Bianchi. Karger, Basel, 1973, p. 1.

137. J. C. Harshbarger. Activities Report, Registry of Tumors in Lower Animals, 1965–73. Smithsonian Institution, Washington, D.C.

138. T. G. Hartley, E. A. Dunstone, J. S. Fitzgerald, S. R. Johns, and J. A. Lamberton. *Lloydia 36*, 217 (1973).

139. J. L. Hartwell (National Cancer Institute), private communication.

139a. J. L. Hartwell. *Lloydia 34*, 386 (1971).

140. J. L. Hartwell. *Lloydia 34*, 221 (1971).

141. J. L. Hartwell. *Lloydia 32*, 153 (1969).

142. J. L. Hartwell. *Lloydia 31*, 71 (1968).

143. J. L. Hartwell. *Lloydia 30*, 379 (1967).

144. J. L. Hartwell. *Cancer Chemother. Rep.*, 19 (1960).

145. J. L. Hartwell and B. J. Abbott. "Antineoplastic Principles in Plants: Recent Developments in the Field," in *Advances in Pharmacology and Chemotherapy*, Vol. 7, Ed. by S. Garattini, A. Goldin, F. Hawking, and I. J. Kopin. Academic Press, New York, 1969, p. 117.

146. J. L. Hartwell and W. E. Detty. *J. Amer. Chem. Soc. 72*, 246 (1950).

147. J. L. Hartwell and A. W. Schrecker. *Fortschr. Chem. Org. Naturst.*, *15*, Ed. by L. Zechmeister. Springer-Verlag, Vienna, 1958, p. 83.

148. Y. Hatsuda and S. Kuyama. *J. Agr. Chem. Soc. Jap.*, *28*, 989 (1954) [*Chem. Abstr.*, *50*, 15522d (1956)].

149. Y. Hatsuda, S. Kuyama, and N. Terashima. *J. Agr. Chem. Soc. Jap. 28*, 992 and 998 (1954) [*Chem. Abstr.*, *50*, 15522h (1956)].

150. L. J. Haynes. *Quart. Rev. London 2*, 46 (1948).

151. E. Hecker and R. Schmidt. "Phorbolesters—The Irritants and Cocarcinogens of Croton Tiglium L.," in *Progress in the Chemistry of Organic Natural Products*, Vol. 31, Ed by W. Herz, H. Grisebach, and G. W. Kirby. Springer-Verlag, New York, 1974, p. 377.

152. C. Heidelberger. "Pyrimidine and Pyrimidine Nucleoside Antimetabolites," Section XIII, in *Cancer Medicine*, Ed. by J. F. Holland and E. Frei, III. Lea and Febiger, Philadelphia, 1973, p. 768.

153. F. R. Heilman and E. C. Kendall. *Endocrinology 34*, 416 (1944).

154. D. W. Henry. *Cancer Chemother. Rep.* Pt 2, *4*, 5 (1974).

155. M. C. Henry, A. R. Roesler, and E. DiDomenico. *Cancer Chemother. Rep.* Pt 1, *59*, 447 (1975).

156. W. Herz. *Recent Adv. Phytochem. 1*, 229 (1966).

157. W. Herz, K. Aota, A. L. Hall, and A. Srinivasan. *J. Org. Chem. 39*, 2013 (1974).

158. E. J. Hessler and H. K. Jahnke. *J. Org. Chem. 35*, 245 (1970).

159. Y. Hirata. *Pure Appl. Chem. 41*, 175 (1975).

160. Y. Hirshaut, R. L. Reagan, S. Perry, V. De Vita, Jr., and M. F. Barile. *Cancer 34*, 1080 (1974).

161. J. S. E. Holker and S. A. Kagal. *J.C.S. Chem. Commun.*, 1574 (1968).

161*a*. J. F. Holland. *New Eng. J. Med. 294*, 440 (1976).

162. C. W. Holzapfel, I. F. H. Purchase, P. S. Steyn, and L. Gouws. *S. Afr. Med. J. 40*, 1100 (1966).

163. E. C. Homes, F. R. Eilber, and D. L. Morton. *J. Amer. Med. Ass. 232*, 1052 (1975).

164. R. Hoover, T. J. Mason, F. W. McKay, and J. F. Fraumeni, Jr. *Science 189*, 1005 (1975).

164*a*. M-T. Huang. *Mol. Pharmacol. 11*, 511 (1975).

165. G. H. Hughes, F. N. Lahey, J. R. Price, and L. J. Webb, *Nature 162*, 223 (1948).

166. T. Ikekawa, F. Iwami, H. Hiranaka, and H. Umezawa. *J. Antibiot. (Tokyo) 17A*, 194 (1964).

167. J. Inagaki, V. Rodriguez, and G. P. Bodey. *Cancer 33*, 568 (1974).

168. E. Iseli, M. Kotake, E. Weiss, and T. Reichstein. *Helv. Chim. Acta 48*, 1093 (1965).

169. N. Ishida, K. Miyazaki, K. Kumagai, and M. Rikimaru. *J. Antibiot. (Tokyo) 18*, 68 (1965).

170. G. W. Ivie, D. A. Witzel, and D. D. Rushing. *J. Agr. Food Chem. 23*, 845 (1975).

171. N. Jaffe and D. Traggis. *Cancer Chemother. Rep.* Pt 3, *6*, 31 (1975).

172. M-M. Janot. "The Ipecac Alkaloids," Chapter 24, in *The Alkaloids, Chemistry and Physiology*, Vol. 3, Ed. by R. H. F. Manske and H. L. Holmes. Academic Press, New York, 1953, p. 363.

173. I. S. Johnson. "Plant Alkaloids," Section XIII, in *Cancer Medicine*, Ed. by J. F. Holland and E. Frei, III. Lea and Febiger, Philadelphia, 1973, p. 840.

174. I. S. Johnson, J. G. Armstrong, M. Gorman, and J. P. Burnett, Jr. *Cancer Res. 23*, 1390 (1963).

175. I. S. Johnson, H. F. Wright, G. H. Svoboda, and J. Vlantis. *Cancer Res. 20*, 1016 (1960).

176. D. F. Jones and S. D. Mills. *J. Med. Chem. 14*, 305 (1971).

177. S. E. Jones. *J. Amer. Med. Ass. 234*, 633 (1975).

178. S. E. Jones, B. G. M. Durie, and S. E. Salmon. *Cancer 36*, 90 (1975).

179. W. F. Jungi and H. J. Senn. *Cancer Chemother. Rep.* Pt 1, *59*, 737 (1975).

180. Y. Kamano and G. R. Pettit. *J. Org. Chem. 39*, 2629 (1974).

181. Y. Kamano and G. R. Pettit. *J. Org. Chem. 38*, 2202 (1973).

182. Y. Kamano, G. R. Pettit, and M. Tozawa. *J.C.S. Perkin Trans. I*, 1976 (1975).

183. Y. Kamano, G. R. Pettit, M. Tozawa, Y. Komeichi, and M. Inoue. *J. Org. Chem. 40*, 2136 (1975).

184. G. Kapadia. *J. Pharm. Sci. 58*, 1555 (1969).

185. H. Kataoka. *Ann. Rep. ITSUU Lab.* (*Tokyo*), 1 (1957) [*Chem. Abstr., 50*, 10113a].

186. W. Keller-Schierlein. "Chemie der Makrolid-Antibiotica," in *Progress in the Chemistry of Organic Natural Products*, Vol. 30, Ed. by W. Herz, H. Grisebach, and G. W. Kirby. Springer-Verlag, New York, 1973, p. 313.

187. W. Keller-Schierlein, M. L. Mihailović, and V. Prelog. *Helv. Chim. Acta, 42*, 305 (1959).

188. R. B. Kelly, E. G. Daniels, and L. B. Spaulding. *J. Med. Chem. 8*, 547 (1965).

189. A. S. Kende, J. Belletire, T. J. Bentley, E. Hume, and J. Airey. *J. Amer. Chem. Soc. 97*, 4425 (1975).

190. A. S. Kende and L. S. Liebeskind. *J. Amer. Chem. Soc. 98*, 267 (1976).

191. J. G. Kidd. *J. Exp. Med. 98*, 565 (1953).

192. K. N. Kilminster and M. Sainsbury. *J. Chem. Soc.*, 2264 (1972).

192a. H. K. Kim, N. R. Farnsworth, H. H. S. Fong, R. N. Blomster, and G. J. Persinos. *Lloydia 33*, 30 (1970).

193. I. Kirson, A. Cohen, and A. Abraham. *J.C.S. Perkin Trans. I*, 2136 (1975).

194. K. W. Kohn, M. J. Waring, D. Glaubiger, and C. A. Friedman. *Cancer Res. 35*, 71 (1975).

195. J. Konopa, A. Matuszkiewicz, M. Hrabowska, and K. Onoszka. *Arzneimittelforschung* (Drug Res.) *24*, 1741 (1974).

196. N. Köriger, D. Živanov, H. H. H. Linde, and K. Meyer. *Helv. Chim. Acta 55*, 2549 (1972).

197. J. S. Kovach, C. G. Moertel, D. L. Ahmann, R. G. Hahan, A. J. Schutt, and J. V. Donadio, Jr. *Cancer Chemother. Rep.* Pt 1, *57*, 341 (1973).

198. G. Koyama, H. Nakamura, Y. Muraoka, T. Takita, K. Maeda, and H. Umezawa. *J. Antibiot.* (*Tokyo*) *26*, 109 (1973).

199. S. M. Kupchan. *Pure Appl. Chem. 21*, 227 (1970).

200. S. M. Kupchan. *Trans. N.Y. Acad. Sci. 32*, 85 (1970).

201. S. M. Kupchan, W. K. Anderson, P. Bollinger, R. W. Doskotch, R. M. Smith, J. A. Saenz Renauld, H. K. Schnoes, A. L. Burlingame, and D. H. Smith. *J. Org. Chem. 34*, 3858 (1969).

202. S. M. Kupchan, Y. Aynehchi, J. M. Cassady, H. K. Schnoes, and A. L. Burlingame. *J. Org. Chem. 34*, 3867 (1969).

203. S. M. Kupchan, R. L. Baxter, C-K. Chiang, C. J. Gilmore, and R. F. Bryan. *J.C.S. Chem. Commun.*, 842 (1973).

204. S. M. Kupchan, R. L. Baxter, M. F. Ziegler, P. M. Smith, and R. F. Bryan. *Experientia 31*, 137 (1975).

205. S. M. Kupchan, A. R. Branfman, A. T. Sneden, A. K. Verma, R. G. Dailey, Jr., Y. Komoda, and Y. Nagao. *J. Amer. Chem. Soc. 97*, 5294 (1975).

206. S. M. Kupchan, R. W. Britton, C. K. Chiang, N. Noyan Alpan, and M. F. Ziegler. *Lloydia 36*, 338 (1973).

207. S. M. Kupchan, R. W. Britton, J. A. Lacadie, M. F. Ziegler, and C. W. Sigel. *J. Org. Chem. 40*, 648 (1975).

208. S. M. Kupchan, R. W. Britton, M. F. Ziegler, C. J. Gilmore, R. J. Restivo, and R. F. Bryan. *J. Amer. Chem. Soc. 95*, 1335 (1973).

209. S. M. Kupchan, K. K. Chakravarti, and N. Yokayama. *J. Pharm. Sci. 52*, 985 (1963).

210. S. M. Kupchan, W. A. Court, R. G. Dailey, Jr., C. J. Gilmore, and R. F. Bryan. *J. Amer. Chem. Soc. 94*, 7194 (1972).

211. S. M. Kupchan, V. H. Davies, T. Fujita, M. R. Cox, R. J. Restivo, and R. F. Bryan. *J. Org. Chem. 38*, 1853 (1973).

212. S. M. Kupchan, A. L. Dessertine, B. T. Blaylock, and R. F. Bryan. *J. Org. Chem. 39*, 2477 (1974).

213. S. M. Kupchan and R. W. Doskotch. *J. Med. Pharm. Chem. 5*, 657 (1962).

214. S. M. Kupchan, M. A. Eakin, and A. M. Thomas. *J. Med. Chem. 14*, 1147 (1971).

216. S. M. Kupchan, T. Fujita, M. Maruyama, and R. W. Britton. *J. Org. Chem. 38*, 1260 (1973).

217. S. M. Kupchan, R. J. Hemingway, and J. C. Hemingway. *J. Org. Chem. 34*, 3894 (1969).

218. S. M. Kupchan, R. J. Hemingway, and R. M. Smith. *J. Org. Chem. 34*, 3898 (1969).

219. S. M. Kupchan, R. J. Hemingway, D. Werner, and A. Karim. *J. Org. Chem. 34*, 3903 (1969).

220. S. M. Kupchan, V. Kameswaran, and J. W. A. Findlay. *J. Org. Chem. 38*, 405 (1973).

221. S. M. Kupchan, A. Karim, and C. Marcks. *J. Org. Chem. 34*, 3912 (1969).

222. S. M. Kupchan, J. E. Kelsey, M. Maruyama, J. M. Cassady, J. C. Hemingway, and J. R. Knox. *J. Org. Chem. 34*, 3876 (1969).

223. S. M. Kupchan, Y. Komoda, A. R. Branfman, R. G. Dailey, Jr., and V. A. Zimmerly. *J. Amer. Chem. Soc. 96*, 3706 (1974).

224. S. M. Kupchan, Y. Komoda, W. A. Court, G. J. Thomas, R. M. Smith, A. Karim, C. J. Gilmore, R. C. Haltiwanger, and R. F. Bryan. *J. Amer. Chem. Soc. 94*, 1354 (1972).

225. S. M. Kupchan and J. A. Lacadie. *J. Org. Chem. 40*, 654 (1975).

226. S. M. Kupchan, A. J. Liepa, V. Kameswaran, and K. Sempuku. *J. Amer. Chem. Soc. 95*, 2995 (1973).

227. S. M. Kupchan, M. Maruyama, R. J. Hemingway, J. C. Hemingway, S. Shibuya, and T. Fujita. *J. Org. Chem. 38*, 2189 (1973).

228. S. M. Kupchan, J. L. Moniot, C. W. Sigel, and R. J. Hemingway. *J. Org. Chem. 36*, 2611 (1971).

229. S. M. Kupchan, C. W. Sigel, L. J. Guttman, R. J. Restivo, and R. F. Bryan. *J. Amer. Chem. Soc. 94*, 1353 (1972).

230. S. M. Kupchan, C. W. Sigel, M. J. Matz, J. A. S. Renauld, R. C. Haltiwanger, and R. F. Bryan. *J. Amer. Chem. Soc. 92*, 4476 (1970).

231. S. M. Kupchan, P. S. Steyn, M. D. Grove, S. M. Horsfield, and S. W. Meitner. *J. Med. Chem. 12*, 167 (1969).

232. S. M. Kupchan, J. G. Sweeny, R. L. Baxter, T. Murae, V. A. Zimmerly, and B. R. Sickles. *J. Amer. Chem. Soc. 97*, 672 (1975).

233. S. M. Kupchan, M. Takasugi, R. M. Smith, and P. S. Steyn. *J. Org. Chem. 36*, 1972 (1971).

234. J. P. Kutney, University of British Columbia, private communication.
235. L. F. Larionov. *Cancer Chemotherapy*, Ed. by W. J. P. Neish. Pergamon Press, New York, 1965.
236. A. I. Laskin and R. S. Robinson. Ger. Offen. 1,904,849, 9/4/69, U.S. Appl. 2/2/68 [*Chem. Abstr.*, *72*, 192 (2155q) (1970)].
237. D. Lavie and E. Glotter. "The Cucurbitanes, a Group of Tetracyclic Triterpenes," in *Progress in the Chemistry of Organic Natural Products*, Vol. 29, Ed. by W. Herz, H. Grisebach, and G. W. Kirby. Springer-Verlag, New York, 1971, p. 307.
238. I. P. Law, F. R. Dick, J. Blom, and P. R. Bergevin. *Cancer 36*, 225 (1975).
239. K-H. Lee, T. Ibuka, H-C. Huang, and D. L. Harris. *J. Pharm. Sci. 64*, 1077 (1975).
240. N. J. Leonard. "Senecio Alkaloids," in *The Alkaloids, Chemistry and Physiology*, Vol. 1, Ed. by R. H. F. Manske and H. L. Holmes. Academic Press Inc., New York, 1950, p. 107.
241. S. Lepetit. *Chem. Abstr. 65*, 1345g (1966).
242. E. M. Lessman and J. E. Sonal. *J. Amer. Med. Ass. 175*, 741 (1961).
243. C. P. Li, A. Goldin, and J. L. Hartwell. *Cancer Chemother. Rep.* Pt 2, *4*, 97 (1974).
244. L. H. Li, T. J. Fraser, E. J. Olin, and B. K. Bhuyan. *Cancer Res. 32*, 2643 (1972).
245. Lissauer. *Klin. Wochenschr. 2*, 403 (1865).
246. R. B. Livingston and S. K. Carter. "Single Agents in Cancer Chemotherapy." IFI/Plenum Data Corp., New York, 1970.
247. R. B. Livingston and S. K. Carter. "L-Asparaginase," Clinical Brochure, National Cancer Institute, Chemotherapy, April 15, 1969.
248. W. Loeffler, R. Mauli, M. E. Ruesch, and H. Staehelin. *Chem. Abstr. 62*, 5856d (1965).
249. C. B. Lozvio and B. B. Lozvio. *J. Nat. Cancer Inst. 50*, 535 (1973).
250. P. L. MacDonald and A. V. Robertson. *Aust. J. Chem. 19*, 275 (1966).
251. T. Machinami and T. Suami. *Bull. Chem. Soc. Jap. 46*, 1013 (1973).
252. H. Maeda. *J. Antibiot. (Tokyo) 27*, 303 (1974).
253. L. Marion. "The Indole Alkaloids," Chapter XIII, in *The Alkaloids, Chemistry and Physiology*, Vol. 2, Ed. by R. H. F. Manske and H. L. Holmes. Academic Press, New York, 1952, p. 369.
254. J. P. Marsh, C. W. Mosher, E. M. Acton, and L. Goodman. *J.C.S. Chem. Commun.*, 973 (1967).
255. E. A. Martell. *Amer. Sci. 63*, 404 (1975).
256. D. G. Martin, C. G. Chidester, S. A. Mizsak, D. J. Duchamp, L. Baczynskyj, W. C. Krueger, R. J. Wunuk, and P. A. Meulman. *J. Antibiot. (Tokyo), 28*, 91 (1975).
257. D. G. Martin, D. J. Duchamp, and C. G. Chidester. *Tetrahedron Lett.*, 2549 (1973).
258. D. G. Martin, L. J. Haňka, and G. L. Neil. *Cancer Chemother. Rep.* Pt 1, *58*, 935 (1974).
259. A. R. Mattocks. *J. Chem. Soc.* (C), 329 (1967).
260. L. E. Mawdesley-Thomas. *Nature 235*, 17 (1972).
261. E. L. McCawley. "Cardioactive Alkaloids," Chapter 39, in *The Alkaloids, Chemistry and Physiology*, Vol. 5, "Pharmacology," Ed. by R. H. F. Manske. Academic Press Inc., New York, 1955, p. 79.

262. J. Meienhofer. *Experientia 21*, 776 (1968).

263. J. Meienhofer, H. Maeda, C. B. Glaser, J. Czombos, and K. Kuromizu. *Science 178*, 875 (1972).

264. W. A. Messmer, M. Tin-Wa, H. H. S. Fong, C. Bevelle, N. R. Farnsworth, D. J. Abraham, and J. Trojánek. *J. Pharm. Sci. 61*, 1858 (1972).

265. A. I. Meyers and R. S. Brinkmeyer. *Tetrahedron Lett.*, 1749 (1975).

266. K. L. Mikolajczak, R. G. Powell, and C. R. Smith. *Tetrahedron 28*, 1995 (1972).

267. N. R. Miller, W. C. Saxinger, M. S. Reitz, R. E. Gallagher, A. M. Wu, R. C. Gallo, and D. Gillespie. *Proc. Nat. Acad. Sci. U.S. 71*, 3177 (1974).

268. M. Miyamoto, Y. Kawamatsu, K. Kawashima, M. Shinohara, K. Tanaka, S. Tatsuoka, and K. Nakanishi. *Tetrahedron 23*, 421 (1967).

269. C. G. Moertel, A. J. Schutt, R. G. Hahn, T. A. Marciniak, and R. J. Reitemeier. *Cancer Chemother. Rep.* Pt 1, *59*, 577 (1975).

270. C. G. Moertel, A. J. Schutt, R. G. Hahn, and R. J. Reitemeier. *Cancer Chemother. Rep. 58*, 229 (1974).

271. C. G. Moertel, A. J. Schutt, R. J. Reitemeier, and R. G. Hahn. *Cancer Chemother. Rep. 56*, 95 (1972).

272. C. Moore, "Synopsis of Clinical Cancer," 2nd Ed. The C. V. Mosby Co., Saint Louis, 1970.

273. S. Moore, M. Kondo, M. Copeland, and J. Meienhofer. *J. Med. Chem. 18*, 1098 (1975).

274. D. L. Morton. *Cancer, 30*, 1647 (1972).

275. Y. Nakayama, M. Kunishima, S. Omoto, T. Takita, and H. Umezawa. *J. Antibiot. (Tokyo) 26*, 400 (1973).

276. L. Nékám and P. Polgar. *Urol. Cutaneous Rev. 52*, 372 (1948) [*Chem. Abstr.*, *44*, 10034i (1950)].

277. N. Neuss, M. Gorman, and I. S. Johnson. "Natural Products in Cancer Chemotherapy," Chapter X, in *Methods in Cancer Research*, Vol. 3, Ed. by H. Busch. Academic Press, New York, 1967, p. 633.

278. T. Nishikawa, K. Kumagai, A. Kudo, and N. Ishida. *J. Antibiot. (Tokyo) 18*, 223 (1965).

279. H. Nishimura, M. Mayama, Y. Komatsu, H. Kato, N. Shimaoka, and Y. Tanaka. *J. Antibiot: (Tokyo) 17*, 148 (1964).

280. N. I. Nissen, H. H. Hansen, H. Pedersen, I. Strøyer, P. Dombernowsky, and M. Hessellund. *Cancer Chemother. Rep.* Pt 1, *59*, 1027 (1975).

281. N. I. Nissen, V. Larsen, H. Pedersen, and K. Thomsen. *Cancer Chemother. Rep.* Pt 1, *56*, 769 (1972).

281a. D. W. Nixon, R. W. Carey, H. D. Suit, and A. C. Aisenberg. *Cancer 36*, 867 (1975).

282. R. L. Noble, C. T. Beer, and J. H. Cutts. *Ann. N.Y. Acad. Sci. 76*, 882 (1958).

283. T. R. Norton and M. Kashiwagi. *J. Pharm. Sci. 61*, 1814 (1972).

284. T. R. Norton, M. Kashiwagi, and R. J. Quinn. *J. Pharm. Sci. 62*, 1464 (1973).

285. M. Novotny in *New York Times*, Dec. 3, 1975, p. 39.

286. A. Ochsner. *Amer. Sci. 59*, 246 (1971).

287. M. J. O'Connell and P. H. Wiernik. *Cancer Chemother. Rep.* Pt 1, *59*, 443 (1975).

288. K. Oda, A. Ichihara, and S. Sakamura. *Tetrahedron Lett.*, 3187 (1975).

289. T. Okazaki, T. Kitahara, and Y. Okami. *J. Antibiot. (Tokyo) 28*, 176 (1975).

290. T. Oki, A. Yoshimoto, Y. Matsuzawa, S. Hori, H. Tone, A. Takamatsu, T. Takeuchi, M. Ishizuka, M. Hamada, and H. Umezawa. *J. Antibiot. (Tokyo)* 28, 479 (1975).
291. P. T. Otis and S. A. Armentrout. *Cancer 36*, 311 (1975).
292. N. A. Pasternak, N. V. Pokidova, V. A. Shenderovich, I. V. Kolosova, and Z. V. Ermolieva. *Antibiotiki 18*, 227 (1973).
293. Pelleter and Caventou. *Ann. Chim. Phys. 14*, 69 (1820).
294. S. W. Pelletier, Ed. *Chemistry of the Alkaloids*. Van Nostrand Reinhold Co., New York, 1970.
295. E. Perlin, J. Engeler, J. W. Reid, J. L. Lokey, and J. Kostinas. *Cancer Chemother. Rep.* Pt 1, *59*, 767 (1975).
296. S. Perry. Reprinted from Seventh National Cancer Conference Proceedings by the American Cancer Society, Inc., *Chemotherapy*, "Cancer Chemotherapy: A Broad Overview." p. 7.11 (1973).
297. G. R. Pettit, private correspondence.
298. G. R. Pettit, unpublished results.
299. G. R. Pettit. *China Quarterly*, in press.
300. G. R. Pettit. "Synthetic Peptides," Vol. 3. Academic Press, New York, 1975.
301. G. R. Pettit and D. S. Alkalay. *J. Org. Chem. 25*, 1363 (1960).
302. G. R. Pettit, M. F. Baumann, and K. N. Rangammal. *J. Med. Pharm. Chem. 5*, 800 (1962).
303. G. R. Pettit, J. C. Budzinski, G. M. Cragg, P. Brown, and L. D. Johnston. *J. Med. Chem. 17*, 1013 (1974).
304. G. R. Pettit, J. F. Day, J. L. Hartwell, and H. B. Wood. *Nature 227*, 962 (1970).
305. G. R. Pettit, J. J. Einck, C. L. Herald, R. H. Ode, R. B. Von Dreele, P. Brown, M. G. Brazhnikova, and G. F. Gause. *J. Amer. Chem. Soc. 97*, 7387 (1975).
306. G. R. Pettit, B. Green, and W. J. Bowyer. *J. Org. Chem. 26*, 2879 (1961).
307. G. R. Pettit, B. Green, and G. L. Dunn. *J. Org. Chem. 35*, 1367 (1970).
308. G. R. Pettit and S. K. Gupta. *Can. J. Chem. 45*, 1561 (1967).
309. G. R. Pettit, J. L. Hartwell, and H. B. Wood. *Cancer Res. 28*, 2168 (1968).
310. G. R. Pettit and C. L. Herald, unpublished studies.
311. G. R. Pettit, C. L. Herald, and D. L. Herald, *J. Pharm. Sci. 65*, 1558 (1976).
312. G. R. Pettit, C. L. Herald, G. F. Judd, G. Bolliger, and P. S. Thayer. *J. Pharm. Sci. 64*, 2023 (1975).
312a. G. R. Pettit, C. L. Herald, R. Von Dreele, M. Allen, L. D. Vanell, J. P. Y. Kao, and W. Blake. *J. Amer. Chem. Soc. 99*, January (1977).
313. G. R. Pettit and L. E. Houghton. *J. Chem. Soc.* (C), 509 (1971).
314. G. R. Pettit, L. E. Houghton, N. H. Rogers, R. M. Coomes, D. F. Berger, P. R. Reucroft, J. F. Day, J. L. Hartwell, and H. B. Wood, Jr. *Experientia 28*, 382 (1972).
315. G. R. Pettit and Y. Kamano, unpublished results.
316. G. R. Pettit and Y. Kamano. *J. Org. Chem. 39*, 3003 (1974).
317. G. R. Pettit, Y. Kamano, F. Bruschweiler, and P. Brown. *J. Org. Chem. 36*, 3736 (1971).
318. G. R. Pettit and R. H. Ode, unpublished studies.
319. G. R. Pettit and R. H. Ode. *Lloydia 39*, 129 (1976).
320. G. R. Pettit, R. H. Ode, and T. B. Harvey, III. *Lloydia 36*, 204 (1973).
321. G. R. Pettit, R. H. Ode, C. L. Herald, R. B. Von Dreele, and C. Michel. *J. Amer. Chem. Soc. 98*, 4677 (1976).

322. G. R. Pettit, R. J. Quinn, T. H. Smith, P. Brown, C. C. Cheng, D. E. O'Brien, W. J. Haggerty, and O. L. Salerni. *J. Org. Chem. 37*, 2789 (1972).
323. G. R. Pettit, P. M. Traxler, and C. P. Pase. *Lloydia 36*, 202 (1973).
324. G. R. Pettit, R. B. Von Dreele, G. Bolliger, P. M. Traxler, and P. Brown. *Experientia 29*, 521 (1973).
324a. G. R. Pettit, R. B. Von Dreele, D. H. Herald, M. T. Edgar, H. B. Wood, Jr. *J. Amer. Chem. Soc. 98*, 6742 (1976).
325. S. W. Pitman, L. M. Parker, M. H. N. Tattersall, N. Jaffe, and E. Frei. *Cancer Chemother. Rep.* Pt 3, *6*, 43 (1975).
326. R. F. Pittillo, M. Lucas, C. Wooley, R. T. Blackwell, and C. Moncrief. *Nature 205*, 773 (1965).
327. J. Polonsky. "Quassinoid Bitter Principles," in *Progress in the Chemistry of Organic Natural Products*, Vol. 30, Ed. by W. Herz, H. Grisebach, and G. W. Kirby. Springer-Verlag, New York, 1973, p. 101.
328. T. C. Pomeroy and R. E. Johnson. *Cancer 35*, 36 (1975).
329. R. G. Powell, D. Weisleder, and C. R. Smith, Jr. *J. Pharm. Sci. 61*, 1227 (1972).
330. J. R. Price. "Acridine Alkaloids," Chapter XII, in *The Alkaloids, Chemistry and Physiology*, Vol. 2, Ed. by R. H. F. Manske and H. L. Holmes. Academic Press, New York, 1952, p. 353.
331. A. Pullman and B. Pullman. *Advan. Cancer Res. 3*, 129 (1971).
332. S. Pyrhönen and E. Johansson. *Lancet*, 592 (1975).
333. R. J. Quinn, M. Kashiwagi, R. E. Moore, and T. R. Norton. *J. Pharm. Sci. 63*, 257 (1974).
334. K. V. Rao. *Cancer Chemother. Rep.* Pt 2, *4*, 11 (1974).
335. K. V. Rao. *J. Med. Chem. 11*, 939 (1968).
336. K. V. Rao. *Antimicrob. Agents Chemother.*, 178 (1961).
337. K. V. Rao, W. P. Cullen, and B. A. Sobin. *Antitumor Antibiotic 12*, 182 (1962).
338. F. J. Rauscher, Jr. *Science 189*, 115 (1975).
339. F. J. Rauscher and T. E. O'Connor. "Virology," Section I, in *Cancer Medicine*, Ed. by J. F. Holland and E. Frei, III. Lea and Febiger, Philadelphia, 1973, p. 15.
340. S. Remillard, L. I. Rebhun, G. A. Howie, and S. M. Kupchan. *Science 189*, 1002 (1975).
341. H. E. Renis, D. T. Gish, B. A. Court, E. E. Eidson, and W. J. Wechter. *J. Med. Chem. 16*, 754 (1973).
342. B. Rensberger in *New York Times*, Nov. 26, 1975, p. 37.
343. B. Rensberger in *New York Times*, Oct. 31, 1975, pp. 1 and 43.
344. J. E. Rhoads. *Cancer 35*, 705 (1975).
345. J. C. Roberts, "Aflatoxins and Sterigmatocystins," in *Progress in the Chemistry of Organic Natural Products*, Vol. 31, Ed. by W. Herz, H. Grisebach, and G. W. Kirby. Springer-Verlag, New York, 1974, p. 119.
346. J. Romo and A. Romo de Vivar. *Fortschr. Chem. Org. Naturst. 25*, 90 (1967).
347. G. Rosen, N. Wollner, C. Tan, S. J. Wu, S. I. Hajdu, W. Cham, G. J. D'Angio, and M. L. Murphy. *Cancer 33*, 384 (1974).
348. C. Rosenbaum and S. K. Carter. "Bleomycin," Clinical Brochure, National Cancer Institute, Chemotherapy, March 1970.
349. S. A. Rosenberg and H. S. Kaplan. *Cancer 35*, 55 (1975).
350. R. B. Ross (CCNSC, National Cancer Institute), private correspondence.
351. R. B. Ross. *J. Chem. Educ. 36*, 368 (1959).
352. M. A. H. Russel. *The Practitioner 212*, 791 (1974).

353. M. L. Samuels, H. T. Barkley, Jr., P. Y. Holoye, P. J. Rosenberg, and T. L. Smith. *Cancer Chemother. Rep.* Pt 1, *59*, 377 (1975).
354. M. L. Samuels, D. E. Johnson, and P. Y. Holoye. *Cancer Chemother. Rep.* Pt 1, *59*, 563 (1975).
355. J. S. Sandberg, F. L. Howsden, A. DiMarco, and A. Goldin. *Cancer Chemother. Rep.* Pt 1, *54*, 1 (1970).
356. W. Sandermann and M. H. Simatupang. *Chem. Ber. 97*, 588 (1964).
357. T. Sasaki and N. Ōtake. *J. Antibiot. (Tokyo) 28*, 552 (1975).
358. U. Schaeppi, F. Menninger, R. W. Fleischman, A. E. Bogden, P. S. Schein, and D. A. Cooney. *Cancer Chemother. Rep.* Pt 3, *5*, 43 (1974).
359. P. S. Schein and S. H. Winokur. *Ann. Intern. Med. 82*, 84 (1975).
360. S. A. Schepartz (National Cancer Institute), private communication.
361. P. J. Scheuer. *Chemistry of Marine Natural Products.* Academic Press, New York, 1973.
362. F. A. Schmid and J. Roberts. *Cancer Chemother. Rep.* Pt. 1, *58*, 829 (1974).
363. B. C. Schmidt. "The National Cancer Research Program," The Robert A. Welch Foundation Research Bulletin, No. 37. Houston, Texas, Nov. 1975.
364. M. A. Schneiderman and D. L. Levin. *Cancer 30*, 1320 (1972).
365. G. Schulte. *Z. Krebsforsch Klin. Onkol. 58*, 500 (1952).
366. M. F. Semmelhack, B. P. Chong, R. D. Stauffer, T. D. Rogerson, A. Chong, and L. D. Jones. *J. Amer. Chem. Soc. 97*, 2507 (1975).
367. S. K. Sengupta, S. K. Tinter, H. Lazarus, B. L. Brown, and E. J. Modest. *J. Med. Chem. 18*, 1175 (1975).
368. M. Shamma and V. St. Georgiev. *J. Pharm. Sci. 63*, 163 (1974).
369. K. Sheth, E. Bianchi, R. Wiedhopf, and J. R. Cole. *J. Pharm. Sci. 62*, 139 (1973).
370. K. Sheth, S. Jolad, R. Wiedhopf, and J. R. Cole. *J. Pharm. Sci. 61*, 1819 (1972).
371. M. B. Shimkin. "Primary Prevention of Cancer," Section V, in *Cancer Medicine,* Ed. by J. F. Holland and E. Frei, III. Lea and Febiger, Philadelphia, 1973, p. 382.
372. S. Siddiqui, D. Firat, and S. Olshin. *Cancer Chemother. Rep.* Pt 1, *57*, 423 (1973).
373. J. D. Skarbek and L. R. Brady. *Lloydia 38*, 369 (1975).
374. B. D. Sklansky, R. S. Mann-Kaplan, A. F. Reynolds, Jr., M. L. Rosenblum, and M. D. Walker. *Cancer 33*, 460 (1974).
375. E. E. Smissman, R. J. Murray, J. D. McChesney, L. L. Houston, and T. L. Pazdernik. *J. Med. Chem. 19*, 148 (1976).
376. P. Smith, W. F. Jungi, C. A. Mayr, G. A. Nagel, and H. Senn. *Eur. J. Cancer 10*, 57 (1974).
377. S. J. Smolenski, H. Silinis, and N. R. Farnsworth. *Lloydia 38*, 411 (1975).
377a. Y. H. Son. *Cancer 36*, 941 (1975).
378. H. Stahelin. *Eur. J. Cancer 6*, 303 (1970).
379. M. W. Stearns and R. H. Leaming. *J. Amer. Med. Ass. 231*, 1388 (1975).
380. J. R. Stephenson, E. J. Smith, L. B. Crittenden, and S. A. Aaronson. *J. Virol. 16*, 27 (1975).
381. C. L. Stevens, K. Grant Taylor, M. E. Munk, W. S. Marshall, K. Noll, G. D. Shah, L. G. Shah, and K. Uzu. *J. Med. Chem. 8*, 1 (1964).
382. C. C. Stock, H. C. Reilly, S. M. Buckley, D. A. Clark, and C. P. Rhoads. *Nature, 173*, 71 (1954).
383. E. J. Stott, M. Probert, and L. H. Thomas. *Nature 255*, 708 (1975).
384. G. H. Stout, W. G. Balkenhol, M. Poling, and G. L. Hickernell. *J. Amer. Chem. Soc. 92*, 1070 (1970).

385. V. V. Subba Reddy, H. N. Jayaram, M. Sirsi, and T. Ramakrishnan. *Arch. Biochem. Biophys. 132*, 262 (1969).
386. G. H. Svoboda. *Lloydia 24*, 173 (1961).
387. G. H. Svoboda, I. S. Johnson, M. Gorman, and N. Neuss. *J. Pharm. Sci. 51*, 707 (1962).
388. G. H. Svoboda, G. A. Poore, P. J. Simpson, and G. B. Boder. *J. Pharm. Sci. 55*, 758 (1966).
389. G. H. Svoboda, M. J. Sweeney, and W. D. Walkling. *J. Pharm. Sci. 60*, 333 (1971).
390. M. Takechi and K. Hayashi. *Biochem. Biophys. Res. Commun. 49*, 584 (1972).
391. T. Takita, Y. Muraoka, T. Yoshioka, A. Fujii, K. Maeda, and H. Umezawa. *J. Antibiot. (Tokyo) 25*, 755 (1972).
392. C. Tamm. "The Antibiotic Complex of the Verrucarins and Roridins," in *Progress in the Chemistry of Organic Natural Products*, Vol. 31, Ed. by W. Herz, H. Grisebach, and G. W. Kirby. Springer-Verlag, New York, 1974, p. 63.
393. D. S. Tarbell, R. M. Carman, D. D. Chapman, S. E. Cremer, A. D. Cross, K. R. Huffman, M. Kunstmann, N. J. McCorkindale, J. G. McNally, Jr., A. Rosowsky, F. H. L. Varino, and R. L. West. *J. Amer. Chem. Soc. 83*, 3096 (1961).
394. W. I. Taylor and N. Farnsworth, Eds. *The Vinca Alkaloids, Botany, Chemistry and Pharmacology*. Marcel Dekker, New York, 1973.
395. H. M. Temin. *Cancer 34*, 1347 (1974).
396. H. Temin and S. Mitutani. *Nature 226*, 1211 (1970).
397. J. Thiemann, Y. Krishnamurthy, S. Murthy, and C. Coronelli. *Chem. Abstr. 71*, 285 (59641d) (1969).
398. R. Thomas, J. Boutagy, and A. Gelbart. *J. Pharm. Sci. 63*, 1649 (1974).
399. M. Tin-Wa, C. L. Bell, C. Bevelle, H. H. S. Fong, and N. R. Farnsworth. *J. Pharm. Sci. 63*, 1476 (1974).
400. M. Tomita, Y. Inubushi, and K. Ito. *Chem. Pharm. Bull. (Tokyo) 2*, 372 (1954).
401. S. J. Torrance, R. M. Wiedhopf, and J. R. Cole. *J. Pharm. Sci. 64*, 887 (1975).
402. A. T. Tu and J. B. Giltner. *Res. Commun. Chem. Pathol. Pharm. 9*, 783 (1974).
403. A. Ulubelen and J. R. Cole. *J. Pharm. Sci. 55*, 1368 (1966).
404. A. Ulubelen, W. F. McCaughey, and J. R. Cole. *J. Pharm. Sci. 56*, 914 (1967).
405. H. Umezawa. "Principles of Antitumor Antibiotic Therapy," Section XIII, in *Cancer Medicine*, Ed. by J. F. Holland and E. Frei, III. Lea and Febiger, Philadelphia, 1973, p. 817.
406. H. Umezawa. *Pure Appl. Chem. 28*, 665 (1971); and a private communication.
407. H. Umezawa, K. Maeda, T. Takeuchi, and Y. Okami. *J. Antibiot. (Tokyo) 19A*, 200 (1966).
408. H. Umezawa, Y. Suhara, T. Takita, and K. Maeda. *J. Antibiot. (Tokyo) 19A*, 210 (1966).
409. J. M. Venditti and B. J. Abbott. *Lloydia 30*, 332 (1967).
410. N. J. Vianna. *Cancer Res. 34*, 1149 (1974).
411. R. B. Von Dreele, G. R. Pettit, G. M. Cragg, and R. H. Ode. *J. Amer. Chem. Soc. 97*, 5256 (1975).
412. A. Von Wartburg, E. Angliker, and J. Renz. *Fasciculus 40*, 1331 (1957).
413. H. Wagner. "Flavonoid-Glykoside," in *Progress in the Chemistry of Organic Natural Products*, Vol. 31, Ed. by W. Herz, H. Grisebach, and G. W. Kirby. Springer-Verlag, New York, 1974, p. 153.
414. S. Waksman and H. B. Woodruff. *Proc. Soc. Exp. Biol. Med. 45*, 609 (1940).

415. M. Wall, American Chemical Society Meeting, Washington, D.C., Sept. 1971.
416. M. E. Wall and M. Wani. International Symposium for the Chemistry of Natural Products (Abstrs. of), 7th, Vol. E138, 1970, p. 614.
417. M. E. Wall, M. C. Wani, C. E. Cook, K. H. Palmer, A. T. McPhail, and G. A. Sim. *J. Amer. Chem. Soc. 88*, 3888 (1966).
418. R. L. Wall and K. P. Clausen. *New Eng. J. Med. 293*, 271 (1975).
419. *Wall Street Journal*, Jan. 20, 1976.
420. *Wall Street Journal*, Jan. 12, 1976; and p. 6, Sept. 23, 1976.
421. E. R. Walwick, C. A. Dekker, and W. K. Roberts. *Proc. Chem. Soc.*, 84 (1959).
422. M. C. Wani, H. L. Taylor, and M. E. Wall. *J.C.S. Chem. Commun.*, 390 (1973).
423. M. C. Wani, H. L. Taylor, M. E. Wall, P. Coggon, and A. T. McPhail. *J. Amer. Chem. Soc. 93*, 2325 (1971).
424. M. C. Wani, H. L. Taylor, M. E. Wall, A. T. McPhail, and K. D. Onan. *J. Amer. Chem. Soc. 97*, 5955 (1975).
424*a*. M. C. Wani and M. E. Wall, *J. Org. Chem. 34*, 1364 (1969).
425. J. S. Webb, D. B. Cosulich, J. H. Mowat, J. B. Patrick, R. W. Broschard, W. E. Meyer, R. P. Williams, C. F. Wolf, W. Fulmor, C. Pidacks, and J. E. Lancaster. *J. Amer. Chem. Soc. 84*, 3185 (1962).
426. A. J. Weinheimer and J. A. Matson. *Lloydia 38*, 378 (1975).
427. J. H. Weisburger. "Chemical Carcinogenesis," Section I, in *Cancer Medicine*, Ed. by J. F. Holland and E. Frei, III. Lea and Febiger, Philadelphia, 1973, p. 45.
428. A. J. Weiss, G. Ramirez, T. Crage, J. Strawitz, L. Goldman, and V. Downing. *Cancer Chemother. Rep. 52*, 611 (1968).
429. H. D. Weiss, M. D. Walker, and P. H. Wiernik. *New Eng. J. Med. 291*, 75 and 127 (1974).
430. S. G. Weiss, M. Tin-Wa, R. E. Perdue, Jr., and N. R. Farnsworth. *J. Pharm. Sci. 64*, 95 (1975).
431. C. Wilhelmsson, J. A. Vedin, D. Elmfeldt, G. Tibblin, and L. Wilhelmsen. *Lancet*, 415 (1975).
432. M. K. Wolpert-Defilippes, R. H. Adamson, R. L. Cysyk, and D. G. Johns. *Biochem. Pharmacol. 24*, 751 (1975).
433. C. M. Wong, R. Schwenk, D. Popien, and T-L. Ho. *Can. J. Chem. 51*, 466 (1973).
434. H. B. Wood (National Cancer Institute), private communication.
435. R. B. Woodward, G. A. Iacobucci, and F. A. Hochstein. *J. Amer. Chem. Soc. 81*, 4434 (1959).
436. E. L. Wynder. *Cancer Res. 35*, 3388 (1975).
437. H. Yagi, O. Hernandez, and D. M. Jerina. *J. Amer. Chem. Soc. 97*, 6881 (1975).
438. K. Zee-Cheng and C. C. Cheng. *J. Pharm. Sci. 59*, 1630 (1970).
439. K-Y. Zee-Cheng, K. D. Paull, and C. C. Cheng. *J. Med. Chem. 17*, 347 (1974).
440. S. Zeisel. *Monatsh. Chem. 4*, 462 (1883).
441. C. G. Zubrod. *Cancer 36*, 267 (1974).
442. C. G. Zubrod. *Life Sci. 14*, 809 (1974).
443. C. G. Zubrod. "Principles of Chemotherapy, Introduction," Section XII, in *Cancer Medicine*, Ed. by J. F. Holland and E. Frei, III. Lea and Febiger, Philadelphia, 1973, p. 601.
444. C. G. Zubrod. *Progress in Clinical Cancer*, Vol. 6, Ed. by I. M. Ariel. Grune and Stratton Co., New York, 1975, p. 73.

Index